Dr. [illegible]

He is ho[illegible] by millions of magazine readers, TV viewers and patients. He is also a man who knows the rewards and difficulties of modern family living.

> "He is *refreshingly nonpontifical* in offering answers to the more than 150 questions included here. Such topics as whining, avoiding homework, playing doctor, teenage dating and seeing the dentist are dealt with in *brief, commonsensical* terms. Salk is realistic in discussing teenage use of marijuana and alcohol . . . He recommends a matter-of-fact attitude about pornographic magazines and birth control pills, noting that changes in sexual mores must be acknowledged . . . his advice (is) *eminently sensible.*"
>
> —*Publishers Weekly*

Other Books by Dr. Lee Salk

What Every Child Would Like Parents To Know About Divorce

What Every Child Would Like His Parents To Know

Published By
WARNER BOOKS

Dear Dr. Salk

Answers to Your Questions About Your Family

DR. LEE SALK

WARNER BOOKS

A Warner Communications Company

WARNER BOOKS EDITION

Portions of this book appeared in a somewhat different form in *McCalls.*

ISBN: 0-446-91486-X

This Warner Books Edition is published by arrangement with Harper & Row, Publishers, Inc., 10 East 53rd Street, New York, N.Y. 10022

Cover photo © Jim Kalett

Warner Books, Inc., 75 Rockefeller Plaza, New York, N.Y. 10019

A Warner Communications Company

First Printing: March, 1980

10 9 8 7 6 5 4 3 2 1

To Juliet Heyer

Contents

Dear Dr. Salk

Introduction

In almost thirty years as a practicing psychologist and university professor, I have been presented with thousands of questions, problems, and situations, touching on almost every conceivable aspect of human relations, problem behavior, and family life. In seeking advice and counsel, my patients and students wanted practical, jargon-free, and scientifically sound information, based on my clinical experience, which would be useful to them in solving their problems. Over the years I've been gratified to learn that my answers and reactions have been helpful to them in achieving greater happiness for themselves, their families, and those of their friends who came into the orbit of these difficulties.

I've found that the question-and-answer approach I've used in this book, which reflects real life situations, is the most valuable and effective. Because the questions and answers have been selected to represent the issues that are of the greatest concern to most people, they will undoubtedly bear on many aspects of your own life. You will notice that the cases presented frequently refer to a person of a specific age or sex; the answers, however, do not always apply solely to people of that age or sex but to a substantially wider age span and usually to both sexes.

There is no logical or meaningful way to organize into sections or chapters the information in this book, and so I have simply listed, in the Contents, the particular problem to which I've addressed my answer. This, together with the detailed index at the back of the book, will help you find what you need to know about your own special concerns.

Spacing Between Children

My husband and I are now thinking about starting a family, and we wonder what the "ideal" spacing between children is. Or doesn't it make a difference?

It does indeed make a difference. Children need a great deal of parental attention in the early years of life, and if this need is compromised, it can affect a child's emotional adjustment.

When children are born very close together, not only are they deprived of the individual care they need but they are inclined to try various and exhausting means of demanding attention. The child—who quickly learns how to harass an overworked parent—also may regard other young siblings as obstacles to the gratification he needs. In turn, the parents, faced with such a situation from day to day, are less likely to enjoy their children, because they have less time and energy.

Some parents have their children close together so they will be "companions"; some do so because they believe that the idea of sharing should be learned early. But although young children can play alongside each other in what we call parallel play, not until the age of three is a child capable of really interacting with other children. Moreover, children between eighteen and thirty months merely grab what they want and are not psychologically ready to grasp the concept of sharing.

I think it's best to keep three years or more between children. By the age of three, a child is considerably more capable of independence, is ready to benefit from a formal educational experience like a nursery school, and has usually mastered two very important developmental tasks: weaning and toilet training. It is also easier to introduce a new member into the family when the sibling is old enough to understand and accept a newcomer.

My husband and I are debating whether or not to have a third child. Our other two children would be quite a bit older than the baby—fourteen and sixteen years older to be exact. Is it fair for there to be such an age gap between a baby and its siblings?

There is absolutely nothing wrong with having such a large age gap between your two present children and your anticipated third child. You can expect, however, some possible embarrassment on the part of your teenagers during your pregnancy. While children in this day and age recognize that their parents engage in sexual activity, your pregnancy provides credible evidence of their mere imaginings. Teenagers are sometimes teased by their peers, and this may make them somewhat defensive. However, I do not consider this to be a problem of any great significance; just be aware that some adolescent awkwardness may occur, and deal with the situation openly.

I do think it is important for you to arrange for genetic counseling to determine if there is any risk involved in your pregnancy. Many people do not realize that the risk of birth defects increases as parents get older, and if you are past thirty-five, you should check with your doctor about any possible complications.

Planning Family Size

When I mentioned that my husband and I were thinking of having another baby (we have three already), my college-age sister smugly delivered her opinion on overpopulation. I didn't say anything, but I felt defensive and angry about her remarks. Isn't it my right to have as many children as we're able to take care of?

I think it is important for parents to evaluate realistically *all* the responsibilities involved in rearing children and to be prepared to make every effort to meet a child's physical and emotional needs. The joys and happiness a child brings are a marvelous reward, but one must recognize that there are also irritations and difficulties.

At the same time, I think it is the responsibility of everyone planning a family to imagine beyond the immediate environment into which a child will be born. We all have, in some way, a hand in the future of the world, and experts have been warning us for many years about the disastrous consequences that may result from overpopulation. Perhaps you might consider adopting a child who needs a home—that too would satisfy your desire to have many children.

If all these aspects have been considered, however, and you and your husband have made a realistic appraisal of your particular situation and motivations in wanting a child, the choice is really a personal one. Tell your sister that you are interested in her opinions and respect them but she must respect yours also. If you verbalize your feelings openly and thoughtfully instead of brooding over her remarks in silence, much of your anger over this matter should be dispelled.

The Only Child

My in-laws say to me, "It's not fair to your baby to be an only child." Is this true? Will my husband and I be risking our three-year-old son's happiness because of our personal desire to have just one child?

I think that it is important for you and your husband to make such a decision yourselves, based on what you feel is right for you. If one child is all you want, I can see no harm whatsoever. The real harm might come if you have a second child simply to provide a sibling for the first. Then you risk feeling conscious or unconscious resentment toward *both* children.

There is no doubt that an only child does lack experiences that siblings have. Obviously, the child who has brothers and sisters must deal with jealousy and resentment, as well as with the pleasures and satisfactions of childhood companionship. A sibling may also have better day-to-day opportunities to learn about sharing—after all, an only child receives considerable attention from both parents and may easily expect this to be the same treatment he will recieve from others outside the family. However, parents can counteract some of these "only-child situations" by making a point of providing opportunities for a child (after he has reached three years of age) to play with others. If your son is encouraged to participate in group activities and is not overprotected by you, he can learn to give and take as well as children do in any circumstances.

Finally, I would like to assure you that there are as many children who wish no siblings had come along as there are only children who wish for a sibling's companionship. Whether a family ultimately decides to have one child or five, there will always be problems—and rewards.

Twins

My first pregnancy resulted in twins, who are now six months old. Everything seems fine, but people have been telling me I must be "careful" or the twins will develop psychological problems. Are they right?

It never ceases to amaze me how intimidating people can be to parents! If you allow yourself to listen, you will even find people telling you about the problems of the older child of twins—and problems of almost any configuration you can imagine. I do not mean to belittle any potential difficulties such children may have but simply to reassure you that in any situation as a parent you are bound to find people whose advice and opinions will arouse your anxiety rather than bolster your confidence.

The psychological problems that twins may develop are basically no different from the psychological problems that any child may develop. The major concern I have about twins centers on the fact that little children require a great deal of time and attention, and when you have twins, it is difficult to give each of them the time and attention that you would have been able to give a single child. Rearing twins obviously takes more time and requires more energy and more ingenuity on the part of the parents. This does not necessarily make twins more vulnerable to problems, but it certainly makes your task as a parent more demanding. By the same token, though, I am sure your joys and pleasures are increased simply because you have *two* children rather than one to provide you with parental satisfaction.

Most people wonder if the identity of one twin will be confused with the identity of the other. If twins want to dress alike, if they are both interested in playing the same games, let them. If they prefer pursuing different interests, they should be given the right to do that, too. The point is to deal with them not as a unit but as two separate people who are developing as individuals.

As I was taking care of my three-year-old twin girls the other day, I realized how easy it is for me to treat them as one. I dress them the same and plop them down with the same diversions. Is it bad for them to be treated so much alike?

It is very common for parents to treat twins as a unit. Feeding them the same and entertaining them with the same games and toys is probably a good idea, since their developmental needs are probably quite similar. If, however, you find that one twin enjoys a particular kind of attention or recreation, I would certainly respect that need and adapt an individual program for her as much as you possibly can without giving in to unreasonable demands.

On the other hand, if both children want to wear polka-dot blouses and green caps, respect that preference, too. In this case, their individuality is being expressed in the same way. Twins should be thought of and dealt with not as a unit but as two separate human beings—even if they both want the same things!

Jealousy and the New Baby

My husband and I are quite concerned about how to prepare our small son for the birth of our second child. Our son will only be twenty months old when the new baby arrives, and therefore too young to understand explanations about why I'm going to the hospital or who the newcomer is. How is it best to treat such a small child upon the arrival of a sibling?

It is extremely difficult, if not impossible, to provide verbal explanations to a child of this age about the birth of a sibling. This is one of the reasons I recommend that parents plan to have children three or more years apart in age.

The matter of deepest concern to a twenty-month-old will be your initial disappearance when you go to the hospital to have the baby. This will seem like an abandonment to your son, particularly if some relatively unfamiliar person comes to take over in your absence. In general, I think it is important for fathers to spend a great deal of time with their children, but it's particularly important at the time a mother goes off to have a new baby. If Daddy is a trusted figure, then the absence of Mother will not create such a void. Ideally, it would be best if your small son could go to the hospital while you are there to see that you still exist and that he has not been abandoned. Unfortunately, very few hospitals allow this kind of visitation, in spite of the fact that it would do much to help an older child adjust to a new sibling.

After the mother's return home, the primary problem lies in helping a sibing deal with a new baby in his life. Clearly, the baby will be very demanding and will require a great deal of the parents' time and attention. It is crucially important that parents recognize that the older sibling still needs undivided time and attention of his own. This parental attention should be given without the child's having to nag, engage in destructive activities, or use some other form of negative behavior to remind you of his need for continued love and affection. It would be wise if you could take him aside to read a book, to go for a walk, or to engage in some activity that he enjoys and that lets him know he is loved as much as before. As he is reassured of your continued love, he will realize that the new baby has detracted in no significant way from his own welfare.

We have a four-year-old boy and a girl who's nearly one. Ever since the baby was born our son has been acting like a baby himself; he crawls around on all fours and talks baby talk; he's also become a terrible behavior problem. Is this the usual way for a child to act?

For a while after the birth of a sibling, a parent can expect an older child to show some "regressive" behavior. By being "just like the baby," the older child may feel that he will gain the same care and attention. But after he has adjusted to the birth of the new one and realized that he is still loved and respected, he usually gives up these temporarily acquired infantile-behavior patterns.

I'm sure your son would not cling to these actions unless they were necessary—necessary to gain a feeling of worth through being "a baby" or through the negative attention it affords him. Because he has persisted so long in this, you may need to seek professional help; but before you do so, try to modify your way of handling him. If you and your husband spend time with him alone on occasions when he doesn't seem to crave it and in a way that you know he enjoys (dragging him along when you go shopping does not count), you will be satisfying the need he is communicating to you. At the same time, the less attention you give to his infantile behavior, the more readily he will relinquish it.

Brothers and Sisters Sharing a Room

We have a little boy, seven, and a girl five. They have always shared the same room—in fact, they've always been close in every way and have resisted any suggestions we've made about moving them to different rooms. We're now wondering though, how long a brother and sister should continue to room together.

There is no hard-and-fast rule about this. In many situations there are no alternatives, because the family may not be able to afford large enough quarters to give each child a room. It is highly unlikely that rooming together will lead to any sexual problems as long as they sleep in their own beds. In fact, studies have shown that when children of the opposite sex are reared together in close proximity, they seem to have less sexual interest in each other and more sexual interest in other playmates who are less familiar. If you find, however, that they are engaging in sex play that goes beyond "I'll show you mine if you show me yours," then perhaps you may want to be more insistent upon changing their sleeping arrangements at this time.

If for some reason you feel that you want them to move into different rooms now, you can give them the incentive to move by encouraging them to help decorate their own rooms with their own things. It is likely that they will want different rooms as they get closer to puberty. At that time, privacy will be so important to them that they will probably request quarters of their own.

Sibling Rivalry

My brother and sister and I are all now married and have families of our own and we're "grownups"—supposedly. But when we're all together at our parents' home, things still come up that make me feel that the other two are more loved and appreciated. Is it right that I still feel twinges of sibling rivalry?

When families unite, it is very common for childhood feelings to arise again. Your feelings may represent the reawakening of some unresolved emotional conflicts. Or it can actually be that your parents *do* appreciate your brother and sister more than they do you. If this is the case, then your feelings are perfectly appropriate and there is nothing you can do about it other than recognize and deal with the fact that your parents, who I am sure do love you, may not love you in the same way as they do your siblings.

Children need acceptance and emotional security from their parents, and when they "grow up" this need is, or should be, gratified by adult relationships. If the transiton is not made, however, an adult may unconsciously continue to vie with siblings for parental attention and approval. If you and this situation is so upsetting that it substantially interferes with your life, or if you are so preoccupied with gaining the acceptance of your parents that you are neglecting your own husband and children, you may need professional help to work through this problem.

The Handicapped Child and Sibling Rivalry

During a family outburst the other day, one of our children announced bitterly that "we only loved and did things for Johnny"—he's our handicapped son, who is ten. It's true, Johnny does get special care, but that's only right, isn't it?

Yes, it is entirely appropriate for you to offer special attention to Johnny, but it is understandable that your other children may feel neglected. This resentment is usually directed more to you than it is to your handicapped son, although it may be displaced onto the handicapped sibling as well.

The best way to handle this is to consider giving the other children undivided attention at times when they don't demand it but would certainly like to have it. The child who arouses concern only when he protests, learns to have fits of anger when he wants something. But if you recognize this need and try to provide gratification of it when everything is going well, the outbursts by the rest of your family should be offset—and your other children will be able to give greater affection to their handicapped brother.

Adoption and Your Children

After being childless for many years, my husband and I adopted a little boy, who is now two years old. Recently, however, I gave birth to a child. As our youngsters grow up, we wonder how to explain the situation to them. We want our older son to feel he's every bit as special as his brother.

Every child, at one time or another, feels that other children are more special than he, particularly if they are his brothers and sisters. Oftentimes this feeling is based on reality: a friend or a sibling actually *is* receiving special treatment because he has achieved recognition in school, because he has an illness or handicap—or because he is adopted. I think it is important to maintain a relaxed, matter-of-fact attitude when situations of this sort occur, dividing parental praise or attention as equally as possible. Otherwise, you may find you are overcompensating and shifting the balance of attention in favor of the child you fear may be left out.

As far as the adoption is concerned: Whenever the timing seems natural and right, or whenever the subject comes up, give your children a frank and uncomplicated explanation. How children respond to this knowledge depends to a great extent on how the whole process has been handled. In my opinion, it is wise to tell a child that a "mother" is the person who has willingly chosen to take care of him and raise him, dispensing love and protection and all the things he needs. In this way it should be clear that the person in whose body the child grew need not be any more important than the person who is actually raising him.

Finally, I think it is important to recognize that children sometimes say things to each other that seem cruel. One day you may hear your adopted child being told by his brother that his own mother didn't want him—but again, if the matter has been talked about openly and you have reassured both children of your love, everyone involved should be able to handle the situation.

Adopting Older Children

My husband and I cannot have children of our own, and we are considering adopting a child. We are wondering about bringing a youngster anywhere from the age of five to ten into our home. Are the chances for success good?

There are so many children in this world who need homes where people sincerely love and want them that I have the deepest respect for you in wanting to make such a child a part of your family.

As long as you are aware of the realities of

parenthood and the potential problems you face, your chances for success are certainly good—but that, of course, depends on what you consider success. If by success you mean molding a child to follow your ways, to adopt all your values and attitudes, and to show love, appreciation, and devotion to you at all times, you are in for disappointment. If, however, you wish to provide a child with a home and an opportunity to develop his or her own resources and sense of self-esteem, you stand a good chance for success.

Unquestionably, early experiences have an influence on later behavior, and some of these effects are irreversible. You must be realistic in your expectations and recognize that a child between five and ten has already had many learning experiences, perhaps under circumstances very different from those in your own life. As a result of this, the child's attitudes, feelings, and values may be quite unlike yours. This does not mean that adopting an older child is a bad or even necessarily questionable idea. It simply calls for more understanding and patience on your part and a greater effort to accept the individuality of that child. As a general rule, it is probably easier if the child you adopt *is* much younger in age—but some of the most challenging experiences in life are the most fulfilling.

Adjusting to a Family Move

Since we've moved into our new home, my three-year-old has had a hard time adjusting. While she used to play happily with old friends, she now refuses even to look at another child. Whenever approached by a would-be playmate, she puts her head down and says, "Go away," and while alone she refuses to try new games or toys. What is wrong? How can I help her accept new friendships and have fun with new activities?

Your daughter is probably very angry with you for taking her away from a familiar environment and bringing her into a new world filled with uncertainties. Children this age consider their parents omnipotent—capable of making almost anything happen, good things as well as bad—and when unsettling events occur, they hold the parents responsible.

The emotional processes of a three-year-old mind are rather fascinating. Your daughter is probably trying to reestablish her old home and her old relationships. By telling new people to go away or by not speaking to them at all, she is reacting as if the move had not taken place. She thinks she can make her former friends come back by not acknowledging the new people she meets. Between being angry with you for causing all this to happen and her attempts to deny it ever took place at all, she must be having a dreadful time.

Perhaps *you* could attempt to meet people who have children her age and arrange a social gathering for all of you. By seeing you interact with the parents of children her age, your daughter may feel safer in reaching out to establish friendships, and the reality of being in a new community may be easier to tolerate. Don't push her in any of this, but do offer her encouragement. I also think you should consider finding a nursery school in your new community. Discuss your problem with the teacher, and see if you can gradually introduce your child to the class over the course of a few visits.

Generally speaking, three-year-olds engage in

activities as a result of "social facilitation." That is, they undertake new activities and experiment with new experiences if they see other children doing those same things. Parents are sometimes astounded to find that a three-year-old who previously responded to calf's liver and spinach with a loud "yuck" is willing to taste the offending food simply because another child eating close by seems to like it. As your child gains a greater feeling of familiarity in her new setting, it is likely that she will want to participate in activities with other children.

Explaining Divorce

After long months of discussion my husband and I have decided to divorce. Now we've got our children to think about—they are six, eleven, and sixteen. Who should tell them, and how is it best to explain what is happening?

Ideally, it is best if both parents do the explaining together, but this is often not possible because there may be strong feelings of animosity between them. In that case, it is advisable that both parents, acting separately, discuss the matter thoughtfully with their children and make several essential points.

The children should be told that their parents have decided they can no longer live together, even though they tried very hard to make things work out. Explaining that "it is better for two people to be happy living apart rather than be unhappy together" helps clarify the decision.

Most children will wonder if they did something wrong or in some way contributed to the breakup of the marriage. It is therefore important to explain to the children that they did nothing to cause this to happen. It is essential to emphasize that, no matter what else happens, "we are still *your* parents —and we will continue to care for you and love you as before."

Children sometimes feel torn because their loyalties are tampered with by one or both parents' jockeying for affection or power. No one can gain from this kind of manipulation—least of all the children. If anything, children are inclined to become anxious and resent a parent who tries to promote bad feeling against the other parent. Throughout the discussion, it should be made clear that both parents are decent people with their children's best interest at heart.

The Absent Father

I was divorced, with a great deal of animosity, when my daughter was less than a year old. At the time her father and I agreed it was best that he never be a part of her life. My daughter is now almost five years old and wondering why she doesn't have a daddy. Could I just tell her he's dead?

No, I don't think you could "just tell her he's dead." Her feeling of trust in you will be seriously at stake if you fail to tell her the truth. It is more than possible that she will eventually learn that she does have a father, and how could she possibly believe anything you say thereafter?

I think it is best for you to tell her the truth in such a way that she does not feel that her father rejected her. Explain that you and her father did not get along and chose to live separate lives. Tell her that at the time it would have been very difficult for both of you to see her without getting very angry with each other. If it is the truth, you should explain that this was very upsetting to him because he loved her very much. If this is *not* the truth, however, do not imply that he had feelings of love but emphasize the fact that he decided it would be best for her.

If I were in your position, I would attempt to contact him and would seriously consider arranging a meeting between your daughter and her father. There is no reason why they can't get to know each other at this time, and it will give your child the feeling that she indeed has a real father who is concerned about her.

Child Custody

After much thoughtful discussion, my wife and I have decided to divorce, and because of the circumstances of our lives, we both agree that I should be the one to have custody of our children, who are eight and eleven. But is this in the children's best interest? Is there a good reason that children should always be placed in the custody of their mothers?

I do not see any good reason for the customary and fairly matter-of-fact procedure of placing children in the custody of their mothers. In fact, I have seen innumerable situations where fathers have been better equipped to meet the children's emotional needs. While the quantity of time parents spend with children is important, the quality of that time is a far more important consideration. Certainly, with mothers spending more and more time away from the home while babysitters and other caretakers tend their children, fathers could act as the "parent in residence" equally as well.

I feel very strongly that parenthood–under whatever circumstances–should be shared equally by father and mothers. Children can benefit enormously from having two parents actively share the responsibility of their emotional and physical welfare; and by balancing this role between father and mother, the parents themselves can gain more freedom without compromising the emotional health of their children.

I think it is essential that we apply the same principle of sharing to divorce situations as we do, or should, in all other parental matters. As the *mutual* responsibilities of child rearing are impressed on parents, perhaps more fathers will be able to gain custody without the mother feeling the stigma of being a bad parent. You and your wife have obviously given considerable thought to this matter and by evaluating your circumstances have come to a conclusion based more on reality than on obsolete convention. Your children can only benefit from such a decision.

My ex-husband and I have both remarried in the last few years. We have a daughter, now fourteen, who has been in my custody until now and who over the past year has been saying that she wants to live with her father. I feel, though, that this is all a whim. Should I simply refuse to let hear make the move?

In situations like this, I feel that children's wishes are a very important factor—and I am speaking for children of all ages. If you are to ignore your daughter's repeated wishes, I am afraid she will begin to see you as an obstacle to her growing independence and freedom. If you accept her choice, you will be in a far better position to provide the kind of guidance you seem to be concerned about. You can help her make the adjustment to a new home and at the same time maintain the kind of good relationship you have with her now.

Whatever her reasons, your daughter does prefer to live with her father. If you interpret this as a personal rejection or if you attribute her motive to overly superficial reasons, she will feel that you are in a sense rejecting *her*, and this can easily cause her feelings of guilt about expressing her true feelings. Why don't you accept her wishes, assist her in making the transition, and give her the feeling that your home will always be open to her and that your love and concern for her will continue as before, regardless of where she lives.

The Stepparent

I recently married a fine man whose first wife died about a year ago; he has children who are now eight through sixteen. There are, however, a number of photographs of the first wife in the house, and many references to her are still made. I certainly don't want to rob the children of their mother's memory, but I do feel that I'm their mother now. How forceful should I be in exerting my own personality in this situation?

I don't think that you should make any effort to influence the children to give up reminiscences or mementos of their own mother. It is perfectly understandable for them still to have these emotional ties to the past; there was obviously a good relationship among the entire family and such warm and tender feelings certainly should not be shut away.

As you become more and more important in your new family's lives, you will find that they in turn will be taking a greater and greater interest in you. In a sense, you will never take the place of their mother—no one can ever really take the place of a lost loved one—and I think that you would be more comfortable recognizing this reality than trying to change it. Remember, these children have spent between seven and fifteen years of their lives with their mother and less than one year with you. Your patience and compassionate understanding in this matter will do much to deepen your relationship with the children.

Conflicts and the Stepparent

I am a recently remarried widow with an eighteen-year-old son. My son and new husband seem to get along just fine, until an argument arises between me and my son. Should my husband get involved in these arguments? Is it his place to discipline my son?

If these arguments do not involve your new husband, I certainly don't think he ought to get involved. If, however, these arguments do involve him, an attempt should be made to talk out all the feelings and issues involved. This principle applies to any family matter, and the fact that you are a widow and he is your new husband doesn't alter that fact.

However, it's important to remember that your new husband is your husband and not his new father. Young people frequently resent a new stepparent because they cling to their relationship with the real parent.

As far as discipline is concerned, it's hard for anyone to enforce rules and regulations on an eighteen-year-old person. With all teenagers and young people, I recommend that parents let these young people know their feelings, desires, and concerns but not attempt to force their own wishes and values on them. If you respect the independence, integrity, and dignity of young people, they will be far more interested in pleasing you and carrying through because of their respect for you. Any attempts to browbeat them, punish them severely, or restrict them arouses antagonism, anger, and rebelliousness and interferes with further communication. This, of course, does not mean that you should have no expectations about your son's behavior. I simply feel that it's important for you to let him know what your expectations and wishes are and let him know how disappointing or discomforting it is if he constantly ignores them.

Stepsibling Jealousy

My family of four children and I, a recent divorcee, will be joining my fiance's family of three children in a few months under one roof. Last week my kids confronted me and said they "hated" their stepsiblings and would refuse to share their rooms in the new house. How can my new husband and I deal with such animosity?

This is indeed one of the most difficult family problems, and there are no easy solutions. While I don't want to be discouraging, I must say that I have encountered some situations similar to this one in my professional practice which caused such strain between the husband and wife that the new marriage was severely jeopardized by the constant tensions, battles, and situations that called for polarization and parents having to take a stand. It's important to remember that each set of children has grown up in a different environment with different parents and has had to abide by different rules and regulations. Bringing them all together under one roof requires major alterations in their lives. It is difficult, if not impossible, for each new parent to take a position other than the defense of his own children when it comes to conflict. Supporting the other parent's children against your own can be very hurtful to your children and can arouse not only jealousy but deep resentment toward you and the new stepsiblings.

In spite of the difficulties I have outlined, I certainly think you should make every effort to resolve this kind of conflict. In my experience I find that by putting young people in the position of having to work out a solution, they frequently come up with workable ideas. If I were you I would gather my children together and explain that you understand their feelings. Make it clear to them that you know that it is difficult to work things out so that everybody will be happy, but you hope that they will make every effort possible to do so. Ask them what they would do if they were in your place. Ask them what solutions they would offer. If they initially take the position "We don't think you should get married in the first place," or "Have his kids live someplace else," then you have to ask them follow-up questions, such as "Wouldn't you like to see me happily married?" and "If you were his children, how would you feel about being asked to live elsewhere?"

While these questions and follow-up questions will not resolve the problem, you will at least be presenting your children with some of the difficulties by asking them to participate in the solution. I suggest you ask your fiancé to do the same thing that you are doing and then perhaps arrange a session where everyone will be together in an attempt to work out ground rules for resolving some of the problems that will arise in adjusting to this new family life.

From time to time you may reach an impasse or find that tempers flare to such an extent that you will need some outside help. I suggest that you seek competent family counseling or family therapy when you begin to feel overwhelmed by these problems.

Perhaps the most important thing to keep in mind is that communication works best when people are in a calm emotional state. When all seems well you can raise some of the potential problems in conversations with your children and explain how much you want things to work out and how much you would appreciate their cooperation. During these times you might find that workable solutions are more easily forthcoming from them than when tempers are up and emotions blazing.

Dating After Divorce

I am the divorced mother of two small children, five and eight. I have recently begun dating and now bring men friends home to dinner with the kids. How can I explain this to them?

Explain it the way it is. To begin with, let them know that you have friends who are grownups, as do all grownups, and that you invite your friends to dinner. Explain that while you were married, their daddy was the person you spent most of your time with, but that is no longer the case. Let them know that you need other people to talk to and be with, and that even though you may enjoy being with other people in no way does that mean that their daddy is not their daddy. Make it clear that these are your friends and that you would like them to be part of your family life from time to time. The fear of most children when this occurs following divorce is that they might lose you. It's absolutely essential for you to make it clear that even if you get to like other people and perhaps even love other people, in no way will that stop you from loving them or make your love for them any less. In fact, point out that when you are happy in your life it makes you a more pleasant person and that you can then share more and more experiences with your children in a pleasant way.

Some children caught up in divorce frequently feel that the parent can only love one person. That results from the fact that some parents interpret the love for one parent as the rejection of the other. This need not be your children's interpretation of your divorce, but unfortunately, when divorce is acrimonious and there is hostility between two people, and an attempt is made by parents to "win" their children over, they frequently feel the expression of love for one parent is equivalent to rejection of the other. This becomes problematical when you begin to date and perhaps become fond of or fall in love with someone, and your children begin to feel threatened. Explain to your children that as they can love both parents, even though their parents are divorced, so too can you love your children and still find emotional satisfaction with a new partner, whether it be a friend or, ultimately, a new spouse.

Single-Parent Dating

I am in my early thirties and have been widowed for about a year, and I am now beginning to date regularly again. My problem is with my children, who are eight and eleven—they are unfailingly and intensely rude to the men I date. Why do you think my children are acting this way? And how should I deal with their antics?

Your children are still clinging, consciously or unconsciously, to their relationship with their father. In their most primitive thoughts, they are still holding out hope for his return and by their rudeness are telling you that they have no room in their hearts for a replacement.

I think it is important for you to discuss this situation with your children at a time when all is well and calm and no one is threatening to disrupt your life together. By talking about their father openly and expressing their feelings of loss, grief, and desire, they will find it easier to accept the irreversibility of the tragedy in their lives. Tell your children that when someone close dies, it is natural to feel sad and lonely. Explain that often people need new friends to make their sadness go away. Tell your children that this is why you go out with other men—and explain that even though no one will ever really take the place of their father, you would like to get married again and hope to find someone who will bring happiness to the whole family. But even while helping them overcome their grief and sadness, I think that you should apply firm and consistent rules that make it clear that their rudeness and unpleasantness are not acceptable under any circumstances.

The Boy Without a Father

I am a thirty-five-year-old woman who has been recently widowed, and I now live alone with my fourteen-month-old son. I have no brothers and my father is quite elderly, so there are few men in my family to help fill my son's life. Does a child of this age miss having a father? And if so, is there anything I can do to make up for this absence?

The relationship between a father and his child is the basis for later experiences that the child will have with males as he or she grows older. If no respected male authority figure is present for a young child, he or she may have difficulty in dealing with the men who are bound to appear in influential positions later in life. A child with only one parent is also denied experiences that would be beneficial: he or she does not see normal warmth and affection being expressed between a man and a woman or hear arguments being resolved in a constructive manner.

While this may seem to represent a somewhat theoretical view of your problem, I feel it is important for you to know these things so that you can organize your life to deal with this situation. By having male friends, you can provide your child with father surrogates and the kind of male figures that can help your child identify with and adjust to male authority. Even though your father is quite elderly, I feel that he can still serve as a father surrogate to some degree. Also, as your son grows older you can encourage his friendship with playmates who might draw him into their family situations. And as time passes, there are sure to be male teachers and friends in your son's life who will do whatever they can to provide him with male companionship and guidance.

Parental Preferences for One Child over Another

My children are four and five. Even though I love and treat them both equally, I'm bothered by the fact that sometimes I find myself "liking" or getting along better with one or the other on certain days. Is it wrong for me to feel this way?

It can be confusing for parents to realize that they sometimes have different and very personal feelings toward each of their children—feelings that vary from mood to mood and situation to situation. In trying to deny these feelings, parents sometimes find themselves plagued by guilt, uncertainty, and a feeling of awkwardness in relating to their children. Face up to the fact you do have ambivalent feelings about each of your children, at times thinking one child is more likable than the other, and at other times finding the likable one altogether irritating. You and the members of your family are all going to go through different moods at different times, and it is perfectly natural that some days you will feel closer to one person than another. The important thing is that you have a basic sense of love and trust that underlies any annoyances or preferences of the moment.

When Parents Break Their Promise

My husband has a habit that upsets me terribly. He's often promising our kids things that he's later unable to follow through on, and then when the anticipated picnic or trip doesn't come off, he's very nonchalant about everyone's disappointment. I think this is quite damaging to children. Am I wrong to be so bothered by something like this?

No, you are not placing too much emphasis on this point at all. In fact, you are quite correct in assuming that this is damaging to children. Promises should not be made unless they can be fulfilled. Apart from the disappointment that this causes the children, it clearly undermines their feeling of trust in their father. An unfulfilled promise is also something akin to a lie; your children can easily get the idea that it is acceptable to say things that are not true. There are, of course, times when plans simply cannot be carried out and a parent must say, "I am sorry. I know I promised it, but it can't be done." But if such irresponsible behavior occurs again and again, a child (or an adult, for that matter) can be made to feel insecure and frustrated.

Like Father, Like Son?

My husband is an excellent athlete and a fanatic about our twelve-year-old son's participation in Little League, school football, and so forth. He insists that Jeffrey take part in such activities, even though it's obvious that our son isn't athletically inclined and would rather read or play a musical instrument. Is this situation affecting Jeffrey emotionally?

I can well understand any parent wishing to share his or her own interests with a child, and I can also understand some disappointment if a child takes on interests that are completely different from the parent's. However, it is crucially important for parents to accept the individuality of their children and help them find those things that offer them the greatest sense of satisfaction.

I'm sure that your son *is* being affected emotionally by this situation. If Jeffrey cannot live up to his father's expectations and if he cannot gain a feeling of being important to his father without losing his own individuality, he may become very rebellious in an effort to establish his independence and may also develop strong hostilities toward his father. Or his self-esteem may diminish; he may come to feel defeated by life and may possibly cope with pressure situations by lowering his levels of aspiration, thus avoiding the anxiety caused by any demands that tax his abilities.

It sounds as though your husband has pushed Jeffrey into the kind of extremely competitive athletic activities that are more adult-oriented than child-oriented. In organizations such as Little League, and even in team sports at school, the emphasis is on winning and not on the joy of participation. I have seen youngsters totally devastated by having made an error during an important Little League event. No matter how much others said, "Don't by upset," the child couldn't be consoled. The child knew how important it was to succeed because he had seen the recognition and the overjoyed adult reactions shown to a teammate whose hit won the game. At all ages children are sensitive and understanding. You cannot convince a child that "winning isn't everything" while at the same time another child is being showered with prizes and congratulations for having won. It is not only unfortunate that your son is under the pressure being placed on him, but it is also unfortunate for his father, who does not seem able to enjoy a relationship with her son based upon the boy's individuality and uniqueness.

The Working Parent

I'm a working mother and it's hard for me to find time for the PTA, the Homeroom Mothers, and a lot of other school-related activities that my kids say the "other mothers" are doing. Is it really important to my children whether or not I get involved in these school activities?

As a general rule, I don't consider it essential for a parent to participate in school activities, but I think that children who have working mothers may possibly feel that their mother's work is more important than they are. Also, your children can easily and understandably get the idea that school is not important if you are not sufficiently concerned to participate.

Children whose parents are too busy to offer positive attention quickly learn that they can arouse parental concern when they do poorly in school, are defiant, or create commotion generally. They are not necessarily problem children—they have, in a sense, problem parents who ignore the emotional needs of their children until the children develop problems of their own. In fact, nothing will work more effectively toward the development of family stress than this sort of emotional configuration.

It is clear that when the working mother cannot participate in school activities, the situation may lead to children's underachievement—or to the development of other types of disruption in their schoolwork. If this happens, your children may be unconsciously testing you to see the extent of your concern or lack of interest in their lives. Their self-esteem is clearly in jeopardy and poor schoolwork may be their message that they need your involvement.

I have been offered a job in the company where I was employed before having my first child, and I intend to accept the offer. My children are seven and eleven now. Is there any special way in which I should prepare them for my new activities in the "outside" world?

Be straightforward about this. Tell your children of your desire to go back to work and assure them that this in no ways means you are rejecting them or do not love them. Your children are old enough to accept this, particularly if they have friends, at school and in the neighborhood who will provide sufficient stimulation in your absence.

You can make your children feel a part of your new life by assuring them that they will see where you work and meet the people you work with. Make it clear that if they are ever ill, someone will definitely be there to take care of them. Also explain that they will be able to reach you quickly if they need you for any reason. Perhaps the most difficult part of all this for children to accept is that they must come home to an empty house. If possible, arrange your hours so that one parent can be there when the children arrive home from school. If not, try to arrange some after-school activities for them, or at least telephone them from your office to ask how things went during the day.

Children's reactions to new situations depend greatly on the kind of emotional investment that has been made in them in the previous years. Children who accept such changes with little difficulty are those whose parents respected them as people and who helped them develop their own individual resources for coping with life"s problems.

My daughter-in-law has announced that she will be going back to work and will be leaving her three-year-old in a day-care center in her neighborhood. But should a young child be left all day in the care of strangers?

Most three-year-olds would find spending all day in this situation too much to handle. Although they are ready for some kind of formal education experience, they still seem to need a great deal of the kind of emotional reinforcement that only parents can provide. The type of child who seems able to develop a greater capacity for deep, warm relationships is the child who is in closer contact with the people who brought him into the world and are strongly motivated to meet his particular needs.

Going back to work can be very important for mothers, but it is essential that a woman's desire to work does not compromise the emotional needs of her child. It is for this reason I advocate, if possible, a schedule that enables the working parent to spend some time in the middle of the day with the child and to be on hand when the child comes home from school. I have seen too many adult patients with substantial emotional problems who have never forgotten the lonely feeling and lack of self-importance that came from returning at the end of a school day and finding no concerned parent there to greet them.

Parental Privacy

I am a parent who prizes her privacy. How can I explain to my three children that I would like a chance to read at least one page of a book uninterrupted by interminable questions? They must learn that my privacy is important, too.

Unquestionably, everyone needs privacy, and that need should be respected. As a general rule, children learn to respect a parent's privacy when a parent is very careful in dealing with the issue of a child's privacy. For example, it's importat for parents not to open a child's mail and to knock on a child's door before entering when it is closed. When you say to a child, "I don't want to interrupt you if you're in the middle of something," you emphasize the issue of privacy and offer your own behavior as a model for how the child is expected to deal with the parent's privacy. It's also important for a parent to explain this process of respecting privacy and, at the same time, to make clear what the specific issues are within that particular family unit. In your case, make it clear that you enjoy reading, require periods of uninterrupted time, and would like that need to be respected. As is usually the case, issues like this are best dealt with when all is well and communication is at its best. This is rarely the case at the moment of crisis and in this case that crisis would be those moments when your privacy is being violated.

It's important to bear in mind that you will probably never achieve your ideal in the form of privacy during your stint as a parent. The commitment of parenthood together with the realities that make up children's behavior—which includes periods of impulsivity and impatience and issues of great urgency—will transcend all the messages and agreements you have between your children and yourself concerning respect for each other's privacy. Taking on the role of being a parent brings with it a certain loss of privacy. In no way can you ever expect to recapture the privacy you and your spouse had before your children were born until they are grown, independent, and living lives of their own away from your home.

Competition Between Parent and Child

My son is constantly bragging that he caught three fish during our vacation and yet I, his daddy, didn't even catch one. This really doesn't bother me now, but I am worried how I will react to his competitiveness in the future when more important issues are at stake.

This issue need not blossom into one of competitiveness, but that depends upon how you deal with it. If it is clear that your self-esteem and feelings for him are in no way altered by his success and that in no way has he detracted anything emotionally from you, then you will have laid a foundation for his being able to accept other people's successes as being issues of individuality rather than one person having greater power over the other. When one person's success causes another person's failure, then the issue of competitiveness can be very intense and color all interaction between two people.

As long as his having caught three fish does not imply failure on your part, you can emphasize how enjoyable it was for both of you to have shared the experience of having gone fishing in the first place and that it gave you great pleasure to see his happiness in succeeding the way he did. The pleasure the two of you have in sharing an experience like this gives him the kind of emotional strength and self-esteem that precludes his having to flaunt his achievements to others as a means of showing his strength and power, particularly at times when he feels emotionally insecure.

Grandparents' Influence on Children's Values

My one-year-old daughter is the only grandchild of my husband's parents, and since we live very close to each other we are together quite often. The problem is that my in-laws are very bigoted and pessimistic people. Are their attitudes likely to affect my daughter?

Children's attitudes are most influenced by the people in whom they have the greatest trust and with whom they have the greatest amount of contact. If your daughter has a warm and trusting relationship with you, it is far more likely that she will adopt your attitudes rather than those of her grandparents. If you ever think she has heard something particularly disturbing from them, however, you could talk with her about it afterward, and explain that you do not agree with what they say. You can also explain frankly to the grandparents that since your views are so different from theirs, you would like them not to express their bigoted views in front of your daughter. If you are deeply disturbed about this, you might even tell them that unless they curtail these expressions, you may be forced to restrict the amount of time your daughter spends with them. Tell them, though, how reluctant you would be to do this, and express hope that they will sufficiently adapt their remarks and attitudes so this need not occur.

Teenage Independence

Our family has been planning a winter vacation all year, and just last month our sixteen-year-old daughter announced that she does not want to go with us and prefers to stay in town with friends. Should we let her?

I think you should certainly encourage her to go along and share in the family's fun. Let her know that you will miss her if she doesn't come and that her presence would probably make everyone's vacation more enjoyable. It's possible that she wants and needs that kind of encouragement in order to be assured that her family wants her along. If you simply take her pronouncement at face value and do not encourage her to come, she may think you didn't really want her anyway. You have nothing to lose by expressing your wish to have her come. However, if she seems firm in her convictions and you feel that she is mature enough to stay back in town with her friends, make sure she has a place to stay, preferably with a reliable friend or relative so that you know where to contact her. It shouldn't be presented to her as a restriction but simply as an extension of your home and family while the rest of you are gone. If she tends to be a morose or unpredictable person and you feel that there is a great likelihood of her getting into difficulty, you should certainly have second thoughts about leaving her behind. This could not only leave her vulnerable to problems but could spoil the family's vacation if something happened and you all had to return.

For the most part, I think any sixteen-year-old who is responsible can be given permission to stay behind provided some reliable friends or relatives offer the structure of their home as a place where she can have her meals, spend her nights, and be with people who would help if any problems arise.

The Teenage Crush

Our fifteen-year-old son has just recently begun spending a great deal of time with our neighbor's teenage daughter, who is a year and a half older than he is. Our problem is that we feel our son may be developing a crush on this girl and we don't want him ultimately to be let down. We also think he shouldn't get involved with a girl older than he is. How can we divert his attentions without hurting his feelings?

There is no way you are going to be able to protect him from the multitude of disappointments he's bound to face in the course of his life. No parent can or should. He's bound to make mistakes. There's nothing wrong with making mistakes because that is the key to learning. In order for a young person to learn to deal with his feelings, which include his feelings of love and his sexual feelings, it's important to be able to have them emerge and to find socially acceptable ways of dealing with them. Obviously, young people need to have some protection from dangers that can lead to irreversible tragedies, but for the most part, it's important for parents to help children develop the resources for being able to cope with life's problems later on.

If the "crush" does lead to disappointment, however, you shouldn't stand by and watch him suffer without offering some guidance and support. Your approach should be one of respect for his assertiveness and individuality. Remember how you would have felt if your parents had said to you, "We know what we're talking about. When you get to be our age then maybe you'll understand what love is, but now you're too young and immature to appreciate it." That statement would have turned you off completely and convinced you that your parents not only did not respect your individuality but had no faith or trust in you either. You should show great understanding for his feelings by letting him know how nice it is to be in love with someone and how hard it is when it doesn't work out the way you want. Explain that he'll feel miserable for a while and as if nothing in the world will make him feel better again. Assure him that while this feeling is real now, it will change eventually. In no way make fun of him or demand the intensity of his feelings or their sincerity. You can be sure that your compassion at that time will go a long way toward helping him learn to love without being turned off by the disappointments that are inevitable in everyone's life.

Teenage Dependency

Our daughter is in her freshman year at college and has managed so far to come home every weekend to visit. We love her dearly and miss her, but frankly my husband and I were looking forward to some time to ourselves for the first time in years, and I wonder if my daughter is having some difficulty making friends at school. She claims she is not homesick and that she does have friends. How can we explain our feelings without hurting hers?

Your problem is indeed unusual. Most parents complain that their children seem to have forgotten them and rarely come home to visit with the frequency they would like. Perhaps your daughter really likes home and enjoys her life there This doesn't mean she is not enjoying college, and perhaps everything she says is true. I see no reason to assume otherwise and wonder why you and your husband can't simply go about your business of enjoying each other anyway. If she is old enough to be in college, in all likelihood she is old enough to be at home alone while you and your husband go off on a trip.

You can simply announce to your daughter that now that she is old enough to be in college you feel she can handle her own needs on her weekend visits at home. If you see her as independent and you feel ready to live your own life without the day-to-day responsibilities of having your daughter living at home, I see no reason why you and your husband can't do what you would otherwise have done if your daughter spent her weekends at college. I certainly don't think you ought to urge her to stay at college so that you and your husband can be alone, That would understandably make her feel rejected.

Exaggerated Teenage Behavior

Our thirteen-year-old daughter has started to use more makeup than a movie star and to dress as if she were a fashion model. She looks ridiculous, but how are we to tell her this and convince her that she would look far better with just a little lipstick?

Young people your daughter's age frequently go from extreme to extreme in testing out their own impact on other people. Accept the fact that she has a need to look sensational in this way and is trying out this kind of costume to see what reactions she creates. Don't try to stop her.

At the same time, let her know what your own tastes are. Don't challenge her tastes but simply accept them as hers and present yours as yours. If it becomes a confrontation, you can be sure she will assert herself in an even more extreme way, which, in all likelihood, is not what either one of you ultimately wants. Trust her and give her the freedom she needs, and you will probably find that she will compromise between one extreme and the other in making this particular choice for her emerging adult identity.

Teenagers and Marijuana

Last week while weeding in the garden I came across what was quite obviously my eighteen-year-old son's stash of marijuana hidden in the bushes. When I confronted him with the evidence, he stalwartly refused to admit that it was his. He is almost entirely independent and will be leaving for college in the fall, so I cannot really punish him or restrict his activities in any way. How can I make clear my concern for his health and safety without entirely alienating his affections?

You can do it by simply stating your concern for his health and safety. Perhaps you would alienate his affection if you made an issue of whether what you found was his or not. Let him know that you are basically not concerned with whether the stash was his, but that you have clear and specific feelings about the possible bad effects smoking marijuana can have on his health. Prepare yourself for the fact that he will, in all likelihood, continue to do what he wants. There is no way you can stop him.

In my experience I find that most people his age smoke marijuana periodically and those who don't are usually the "goody-goodies" who are not among the better-adjusted young people. I am not suggesting that smoking marijuana is a sign of maturity, but it's important to take into consideration those activities among young people that represent a current trend. All young people try out things that are considered unacceptable in their search for independence. Many of them simply try things to feel they've done it and simply stop at that. Others, perhaps with weak family ties or underlying feelings of inadequacy, seem to go from one self-destructive thing to another.

Don't hesitate to let your son know how much you love him and that even when he does things that are unacceptable, which upset and annoy you, you still love him and will help him if he ever gets into any difficulty or has any problems. Parents frequently make a mistake by saying, "If you continue to do things, I disapprove of, then you can just go out into the world—forget all about me and don't even come to me when you need help!" While this may represent your feelings at that time, you would be very upset if he took you at your word and left. No one wins when a conflict is resolved in that way.

Teenage Drinking

My fifteen-year-old daughter came home the other evening from a party reeking of alcohol and barely able to keep her balance. I was horrified and told her that she would not be allowed to attend another party for six months. She answered that if she wanted to drink, she could do it anywhere and anytime—not just at parties. I'm afraid that this is true. What's to be done?

She is absolutely right—if she wanted to drink she could probably do it anywhere and not just at parties. What she is saying is that she is in a position where she can actively defy you. She is also telling you she resents the severe restrictions you are placing on her.

While I can understand your being upset with her, look at it from her viewpoint. She will be deprived of her social life at an age when it is extremely important for young people to be with their friends. Moreover, she will probably find it embarrassing to face her friends and let them know she can't socialize with them for six months. Her anger and resentment toward you can indeed motivate her to get back at you and show you that she can do what she wants despite your restrictions. If you pursue this course, in all likelihood you will be faced with a series of head-on confrontations where you not only stand the chance of losing face and losing your authority but where she can also lose her respect for you. This, of course, is not to mention the fact that she will not be learning the lesson you are trying to get across, but she will learn instead that she can do what she wants in ways over which you have no control.

I believe it's important for you, as a parent of a teenager, to let your views on these issues be known. Prepare yourself for the fact that your child may ignore your warnings and even do the opposite of what you say from time to time. This is the teenagers' way of asserting themselves in an attempt to achieve independence and individuality. If you think back in your own life to those teenage years, I am sure you will find that you had a tendency to do the same thing with your parents. Remembering your own parents' responses may give you greater insight and help you find the best approach to handling your daughter and her problems now.

Perhaps you ought to reconsider what you did with your daughter and tell her that you have reconsidered your punishment and feel that it would be unfair to restrict her from parties. Tell her you were very upset by seeing her drunk and that this caused you to set that restriction. Explain to her that you know that she can drink at times other than parties and in all likelihood can do whatever she wants. Let her know there is basically no way you can stop her but that you want her to know that you love her a great deal, are deeply concerned with her welfare, and would be very upset and disappointed if she were to repeat this incident. Make it clear that while she can do what she wants, she can in fact get herself into a great deal of difficulty, not to mention all the physical hazards that are involved in drinking alcohol.

The basic point for you to get across to your

daughter is that she is independent and an individual and that you respect her individuality, but you have feelings about what she is doing and you want her to know how you feel. If you have had a trusting and close relationship with her in the past, in all likelihood she will be concerned about your reactions to her. Despite the defiance and rebelliousness I've seen from teenagers, I'm also aware of the fact that they want parental acceptance and love. If you respect their individuality, even recognizing the hazards that are involved in giving them the freedom they need, there is less of a chance for them to defy you in self-destructive ways, Don't lose sight of the fact that she is at an age when you cannot police her all of the time and there is no way you can prevent her from making mistakes. Not only don't I recommend policing any young person all the time, but I believe that with an open relationship between a parent and a young person, you can guide them more effectively and help them learn by their mistakes. What's most important is that they need freedom in order to learn and one learns by making mistakes. As long as you are in a position where there is mutual respect you can be a very effective guide to your teenager during this potentially stormy period.

Defiance of Parents

My teenager and her date (both freshmen in high school) announced that they were off to see a movie that I know from the reviews to be tasteless and sadistic. I told them they couldn't go, and the evening ended in an uproar. Is it wrong for me to act as censor?

I think it is essential for parents to convey their thoughts and ideas to their children, particularly to adolescents. However, expressing opinions is one thing; insisting on their acceptance is another. In fact, one can predict with certainty that an adolescent will reject his parents' ideas and turn to opposing ones—it's part of the normal pattern in our culture through which the adolescent establishes his identity and self-esteem.

Because of this whole complicated adolescent process, I think it would be best if you expressed your sincere reactions about the movie—being quick to mention that you haven't seen it but have heard of its content—and offer another choice. If you take a very strong stand against the film, you can make it seem more intriguing than it really is and motivate the young people to see it out of defiance. On the other hand, if you express no concern, you are giving them no guidelines by which they can assert themselves as individuals. So let your feelings be known, but without insisting that your wishes be followed.

The Introverted Teenager

We worry about our fourteen-year-old daughter—she's always been in the shadow of our older daughters, whose ages range from eighteen through twenty-three and who are outgoing and very popular. Our fourteen-year-old seems much more withdrawn and not particularly interested in cheerleading or dances or any of the other activities that her sisters always enjoyed. We're concerned. Is something the matter?

It sounds as though your fourteen-year-old daughter simply has a different temperament; she sounds more introspective and introverted. But this doesn't mean she is any less happy than her sisters, who are extroverted and involved. I'm sure you realize that some people enjoy talking and other people enjoy listening, that some want to perform while others want to watch, and each of these personality types gains her own kind of pleasure and satisfaction from her experiences.

As the youngest child in a succession of outgoing sisters, however, your fourteen-year-old may be comparing herself with the others—or feel that you are making such a comparison. Children are very sensitive and often respond to their parent's values in perplexing ways. Your daughter may be responding to subtle pressures on your part that even *you* are not aware of. Your well-meaning "concern" may be interpreted by her as a devaluation of her own personality, or of her social or academic inclinations.

I think that you should accept your daughter's individuality, and praise and encourage her in what she does best. Make a concerted effort to find out what her interests are. She may be somewhat withdrawn in expressing her feelings if she senses that you tend to approve the kind of interests that her older sisters have had; and she may fear your disapproval if she expresses any divergence from this family "pattern." Avoid at all costs conveying the idea that there is something "wrong" with her because she is not following the trend that her older sisters have set. And eventually you may find your daughter to be the personification of the expression "still waters run deep!"

Teenage Withdrawal

My fourteen-year-old daughter has recently developed a pattern of staying by herself in her room during most of her free time. She seems perfectly happy, but all she ever wants to do is listen to records by herself or read. Is this withdrawal from us a normal stage of development?

It is not at all uncommon for adolescents in our culture to show a marked change in behavior during puberty. At this time in their lives, they are struggling to assert themselves and to establish their independence; they are experimenting with different ideas and philosophies and they fantasize about the future. If your daughter is indeed perfectly happy and shows no signs of depression, distress, or bizarre behavior, it is more than likely that she is going through a normal stage in her development.

If she seems depressed and under pressure most of the time, you might want to find a psychologist or psychiatrist who specializes in the counseling of adolescents, simply to give her the opportunity to talk with someone who is not part of her immediate family. By doing so, you would be offering her help if she needs it and at the same time reassuring yourself that there are no underlying emotional disorders.

The length of time it takes an adolescent to come out of this stage varies. Sometimes it's a matter of weeks, sometimes months, and in rare instances a year or more. Perhaps the best thing for you to do is to accept this as a normal developmental stage—eventually to be replaced by some other stage that may be equally baffling.

Teenage Shyness

My eighteen-year-old daughter is attractive and healthy, but she is not dating and never has. She's a bookworm and very shy—but she also seems happy. Should I be worried that she's not as interested in boys as other girls are?

It is my feeling that you should leave her alone and let her continue to be happy the way she is. Perhaps, in a moment when you are having a conversation and feel close, you could ask her—in a completely uncritical way—why she doesn't seem interested in boys. You may find that she is simply more interested in books and ideas at this time. Or perhaps she will indicate that her shyness prevents her from dating, and then you can offer her your reassurance and support, or even professional help if you sense it is needed. In any event, don't worry about it. If you find that she has a sensible and realistic attitude and is not unduly disturbed by the situation, leave her alone in her contentment.

Respecting Your Child's Privacy

While going through my teenage daughter's drawers, I discovered a letter from a girl friend who had moved away. When I later referred to something I had read in the letter, my daughter became infuriated that I had been going through her things. Is she being unreasonable, or am I?

Your daughter has every right to feel angry. Children of all ages need to have some degree of privacy, and when they are teenagers they certainly require more. While teenagers in our society are inclined to react intensely to any of their feelings, your daughter's reaction would be understandable at any age. How would you feel if she referred to some matter in your life that you had no intention that she know? Needless to say, you would feel angry, possibly humiliated, and suspicious that she might do this again.

Try to set things straight by apologizing for what you have done. Explain to your daughter that you have given the matter more thought and realize that she was right—and tell her that you will not violate her privacy again.

Meddlesome Parents

I am a sixteen-year-old-girl, and I have a mother who insists on ruling my life. She and my father were divorced four years ago, and since then my mother has "attacks" and "fainting spells" if I date people or have friends she doesn't approve of. The doctor says there's nothing the matter with her, but I get scared. And I get angry too. Why does my mother act like this?

Your mother undoubtedly is an unhappy woman, and events in her life obviously have not worked out to her satisfaction. If, as the doctor says, there is nothing wrong with her, then your mother's fainting spells and attacks are attempts to control you—to make you feel guilty for causing them by your behavior.

This is a very primitive way of trying to control others, and I can certainly understand your feelings of fear and anger. Her actions cannot possibly help you to function in a healthy way. I'm sure you find it difficult to make decisions without being terribly influenced by how your mother will react; perhaps you have been greatly tempted to deceive your mother in order to avoid conflict; and perhaps you have even tried to get back at your mother by doing things neither of you approve of.

It seems advisable to speak to your doctor and ask that he arrange for your mother to get appropriate psychological or psychiatric help. I also urge that you speak with the doctor about *your* feelings; if he cannot help you come to terms with your dilemma, he should suggest a counselor who can.

Respecting Teenage Privacy

My fifteen-year-old daughter is friends with a very nice boy from her class at school, and the two of them will often study together in her room with the door closed. Should I insist that the door be left open?

You might casually mention to your daughter the possibility of leaving her door open while she and her friend study. But if she says that she wants the privacy of a closed door, I think you should respect her wishes. Frankly there is no way to force this issue without conveying the idea that you don't trust her—and it would be understandable for her to be both defensive and resentful about this. If you do trust your daughter and have been honest in discussing reproduction and sex with her, she undoubtedly understands the implications of being alone with a boy under these circumtances. For you to suggest, however, that sexual activities always occur when people are behind a closed door is in itself a provocative idea. Remember, whatever she can do in her room, she can do elsewhere anyway. It is far better for her to feel welcome in her own home than it is to institute a strict "open-door policy" for no real reason.

It sounds to me as if she has a good relationship with this boy, and if they are studying together and doing well in school, I see no cause for alarm. The most important thing is to maintain a trusting relationship so that your teenager can come to you with any problems and questions she has and to give her enough freedom so that she can develop a sense of responsibility for her own actions. If you stifle her and restrict her, you will only drive her away and prevent her from basing her own set of values on your guidance.

Dressing Like the Other Kids

My daughter comes home whining every day that she is the only one in the class who doesn't wear high-heeled shoes. I don't think she is old enough to wear them, but this silly little disagreement is causing a major battle in our home. What should I do?

While this disagreement may seem silly to you, it may be far more complicated than it seems superficially. If you look back into your own youth, you will find that when your best friend had something or did something you may have felt a great internal pressure to do the same thing in an effort to gain recognition and acceptance by that friend. From your point of view, at that age, the "whole world" was doing it, and that was the basis of your appeal to your parents. From your point of view, your best friend can be your "whole world." You may also have feared embarrassment if you did not conform to what your best friend or best friends were doing. These are realities that are very intense and important in the lives of young people.

Parents need to be compassionate when children express wishes in this way, but I *don't* believe that parents should allow other children to run their lives or their homes. If you feel strongly about high-heeled shoes on a child—and I can easily understand your feelings—make it absolutely clear that under no circumstances will you buy or allow your child to wear them. Assuming that for the most part your child and you see eye to eye on other issues and that you have complied with her wishes for a good part of the time, simply make it clear this is one issue you feel strongly about and no one will budge you. Show that you know she disagrees and that it will hurt her feelings but that she will unfortunately have to learn to live with that dissatisfaction on this issue. Tell her that she can explain to her friends that her parents just don't share her feelings about high heels, and if she wants to consider it meanness on your part, to feel free to explain to her friends that your insistence is unalterable.

Let her know that you understand her desire to do the things her friends do, but that you have no intention of letting them set your values, any more than you intend to comply with all the regulations their parents set on their behavior. I'm sure some of her friends have earlier bedtime than she or perhaps have more responsibilities around the home than she. Let her know it would be as unreasonable for you to impose the restrictions they've applied to their children on your child as it would be for you to allow them to decide what clothes you will buy and allow her to wear.

Keeping "Bad" Company

My thirteen-year-old daughter is sweet but still rather immature and quite impressionable. The girls she's been spending time with lately, though, seem fairly sophisticated and do things of which my husband and I don't approve: they smoke and have dates and move in a fast sort of crowd. Am I wrong to think that my daughter will be affected by these companions?

Your daughter is approaching an age when it will be extremely difficult—and at times impossible—to control all her choices and actions. At the same time, she is entering a stage in which she will do her best to assert herself and show how independent and responsible she can be. This creates a paradoxical and perplexing situation for parents. On the one hand, adolescents need freedom to develop and demonstrate their sense of responsibility, but, on the other hand, they are still relatively immature, and their new-found freedom can be too much for them to handle.

I think it would be best for you to maintain warm and open communication with your daughter and show respect for her ideas and values, whether or not they correspond with your own. Do, however, let her know your feelings and, in an uncritical and low-key way, make it clear what it is you approve or disapprove of. Emphasize that you fear that she might be drawn into situations that would make you unhappy. Encourage her participation in activities that give you more peace of mind while at the same time allowing her to function independently as an individual in the context to these new experiences.

True, you could simply forbid your child to see these girls. However, many teenagers tend to be assertive and rebellious and inclined to do precisely what you forbid them to do. In the ensuing dispute, you run the risk of losing communication with them altogether.

While such friends do have an influence on young people, the important relationship is the one children have had with their parents throughout the years. If you have been honest with your daughter and maintained a relationship of trust and love, she will in all likelihood be much more impressed by your values than those of her peers.

Teenage Hero Worship

My thirteen-year-old daughter has a violent "crush" on the male star of her favorite television program. She's learned every detail of his life, composes letters to him, imagines going to his home to meet him. Is it normal for youngsters to have such fantasies about TV stars? Her interest in him seems all-consuming—and this has been going on for months now.

It is not at all uncommon for young people to become attached to a star. Identification with such a person helps children to develop their own identities and define their own aspirations.

In order for your daughter to establish relationships with people her own age, both male and female, she must relinquish some of her ties with her parents. This transition takes place as she shifts her admiration and all-consuming interest to someone outside her home. If you recognize that the idealization of a hero is a step toward a child's independence and individuality, you may find this situation easier to tolerate. In any event, do not make fun of your daughter—her feelings are very real and important to her.

Teenage Vandalism

A teacher recently saw our thirteen-year-old son and two other boys twisting off the windshield wipers and radio antennas of several cars in the school parking lot. Even though the incident was a relatively minor one, and our son seemed quite remorseful about his part in it, we are still quite upset. Why would thirteen-year-old boys do such a thing? Is this an indication that there is something emotionally wrong with our son?

If this is an isolated instance of destructive behavior about which your son feels genuine remorse, it is not likely that it represents any underlying emotional problem. Youngsters of this age engage in a certain kind of rebelliousness as part of a normal attempt to express their individuality. At this age, they not only want more independence, but they also feel they can handle it. Their efforts to prove their own abilities often result in a defiance of authority. Children your son's age are also susceptible to peer pressure and may "go along with the group" just to be accepted. To a certain extent, all this is normal, but if these factors continue to manifest themselves in antisocial behavior, it does represent an emotional problem.

Your son's remorse is a good sign. It means he has a conscience and a concept of right and wrong. You should now impress on him the fact that he has destroyed property and committed an act that could get him into serious trouble. While showing your deep concern about this incident, and at the same time making clear the possible consequences of his act, try to create an atmosphere in which he can talk about the episode and describe how it came about in the first place. His response may give you some more clues for the reason behind his action. Some children who feel neglected or who feel their parents pay attention to them only when they get into trouble are more inclined toward vandalism than are children who gain a sense of self-esteem through more acceptable behavior.

I think it is only fair that your son offer reparations to those people whose cars were damaged. Urge him not only to apologize but also to pay for the repairs with his own money; this will help him feel a greater sense of responsibility for his behavior. If he has no funds, help him find opportunities to earn the money. In this way you will be expressing your disapproval of his act and offering support to him in undoing the damage. Furthermore, this will help him gain a sense of self-esteem and independence through a positive gesture rather than through a negative act.

Teenage Dating

My fourteen-year-old daughter has recently acquired a boy-friend, whom she goes to baseball games and teenage dances with. My husband thinks this is cute, but I don't know if we should encourage it. How old should a teenager be before she starts seeing one person exclusively?

It is hard to establish a specific age when this sort of thing is right or not right, since so much depends on the youngster's maturity and personality. I can best answer this question not by giving you any set rule of age to follow but by advising you to focus on a greater understanding of your daughter as an individual.

In many ways, your daughter is demonstrating a capacity to relate well to one person, and if she seems to be enjoying such close companionship, it can be a positive experience. I don't think you or your husband should openly try to control what she is doing. But if you make every attempt to keep channels of communication open, she should feel free to discuss her feelings about her boyfriend with you. In this way, you can help her use her own resources to keep the relationship in perspective and to deal with whatever problems may come up.

As teenagers struggle for independence and an identity of their own, they may sometimes do the opposite of what their parents wish simply to show their own individuality. All too often I have seen teenagers cling to a relationship with another person simply because parents objected to it. For this reason, it is best not to raise strenuous opposition to her dating unless what she is doing is clearly self-destructive.

I can also assure you that it is perfectly normal for teenagers to suppose that their love of the moment is the one they will want forever; do not be shocked if before long someone else becomes the "love forever" of your youngster's life.

Automobiles and Teenagers

Our daughter will soon be sixteen, and most of the young people her age in our suburban community are allowed to have their own automobiles. We can afford to give her a car, but should we? Should teenagers have such lavish presents?

It is impossible to draw a line at the point where presents for teenagers become too lavish. Much of the answer depends upon the parents' values, the community the family lives in, and the peer pressures the youngsters are under. In your particular circumstances, it would seem normal for *your* teenager to have a car.

My main concern, however, is that a teenager develop a sense of responsibility about having an automobile. I think that you must discuss carefully and lay down firmly the rules and regulations that are appropriate for the use of a car. While you may be economically able to buy a new or used car outright, I think it would be a more meaningful experience for your daughter if she were to contribute to the cost of it. If she is old enough to drive the car, then she should be able to get a job to help finance the cost.

Pornography and Your Teenager

While cleaning up my thirteen-year-old son's room, I discovered in the back of his closet a cache of "girlie" magazines and even some hard-core pornography. How much of a fuss should I make over this?

I don't think you should make any fuss at all. In attempts to come to terms with their own sexuality, it is very common for teenagers to show curiosity about various kinds of sexual information. And while many people may continue to harbor some interest in pornography, their interest seems to diminish because it has been satiated rather than suppressed.

Parents should take a matter-of-fact attitude. At the same time, you could point out that it's bad taste to tack it on the walls or put it among the other magazines for family reading. Also, without preaching, you might give your opinion that pornography illustrates only one aspect—and often a small and drastically distorted aspect—of normal sexual activity.

How a child copes with exposure to pornography really depends on how parents have dealt with the child's sex education. If information about sex has been dispensed honestly and in a healthy context, then less wholesome aspects of sex should assume their proper perspective in a youngster's mind.

Problems of Adjustment Beyond Adolescence

After getting out of the army, our twenty-two-year-old son asked if he could move back in with us "until he got oriented and decided what he wanted to do." We're glad to have him around, but months are passing and he doesn't seem to have any sense of direction about his future. Should we be pressuring him to get on with a life of his own?

I think it is important for your son to feel accepted at home and for you to cultivate a trusting relationship with him so he can openly discuss his feelings.

I don't think you should give him a deadline or pressure him to leave, but I do think you should urge him to begin exploring possiblities for a life of his own. Ask him to give serious thought to the kind of thing he wants to do or try out while he is still living with you. Talk to him about interests or activities that give him satisfaction and a feeling of fulfillment. If you encourage him in this kind of exploration, the realities of life will become more a part of his everyday existence at home. Once he begins to develop his life in a given direction, I see no harm in his staying at home until his activities and plans become firmer. Then when he has achieved that degree of independence, he may express an interest in living away from your house. If he does not offer to move, you could suggest that he might enjoy the privacy of his own living quarters. If all of this is done in a loving and supportive way, he should have no feeling that he is being rejected.

I'm a nineteen-year-old girl and I'm still living with my parents. I've been working ever since I graduated from high school, and now I feel that I'd like to move into an apartment of my own here in the same city. My parents are horrified. They act very hurt whenever I mention the subject. Why do they react this way? Is it wrong for me to want a place of my own?

I do not think that it is at all wrong to want a place of your own. Many parents are distressed at this thought, partly because they grew up in a different era. There was a time when parents interpreted a child's move away from the family as a rejection or as an indication that he or she was about to engage in an "illicit" form of social life. As reassuring and responsible as you may be, it is sometimes hard for parents to accept the fact that their child is now an adult able to function on his or her own.

It is a shame that parents are constantly trying to get their children to show a sense of responsibility and freedom and yet keep preventing them from doing so. I have in the past felt that parents react this way because they forget what it was like to be nineteen years of age, but I now think it may very well be the opposite—they may *remember* what their feelings and desires were and are fearful that you will have the same impulses and wishes they had. Another explanation may be that they want you to be dependent on them because they enjoy the roles of mother and father. They may find it too much of an adjustment to go back to being primarily husband and wife again. This often happens in a marriage where people do not get as much satisfaction from each other as they do from their children, causing them to react with alarm at the idea that their children are growing up and moving out into the world.

But regardless of their reasons, I think it is important for you to take this step toward independence. While your parents may not like it, they must learn to accept it.

When our oldest daughter came home from her freshman year at college, one of the first things she did was light up a cigarette. Her father was furious that she had taken up smoking, and the two of them have been having terrible arguments about it ever since. He tells her how bad it is for her health, and she seems to agree—yet she says that she has a right to do what she wants. Should my husband keep nagging her about this? I don't like it either, but I don't see how you can forbid a child of this age to smoke if she wishes.

You are absolutely right—you can't prevent a child of this age from doing most things she wants to do. I can well understand her father's feeling—he is concerned about his daughter's health and recognizes the real hazard that smoking is. At the same time, it is equally important for him to recognize that his daughter has the right to do whatever she wants at this stage in her life, whether he agrees with it or not.

I don't think continued nagging will have any positive effect whatsoever. In fact, your daughter may smoke all the more defiantly in order to assert her independence. Your husband would be far better off if, after making his position clear, he told her she is now old enough to decide how she wants to treat her own body and leave it at that. If he is less emotional about the subject, she may be more inclined to modify her behavior on the basis of her own knowledge that smoking is bad for her health. In a sense, both daughter and father are caught up in an emotional whirlpool. By neutralizing the emotional aspect of the conflict, the issue of smoking itself—rather than the *right* to smoke—becomes predominant, and your daughter's own common sense will probably prevail.

We're worried about our daughter, a lovely and seemingly well-adjusted young woman of twenty-eight who has had several marriage proposals—but has refused them all because the man "isn't the right person." The rest of us kid her about being so particular, but actually her father and I are a little worried. Isn't there something the matter when a person has such high standards? I wanted to marry my husband when I was nineteen.

I am sure you would agree that it is far better for your daughter to continue being content in her single life than it is to marry someone just for the sake of marrying. She is far better off following her *own* standards of what she wants rather than accepting other people's criteria about the "right" person and the "right" life style.

True, there are people so demanding that they will become involved only with certain people who have specific characteristics; they are looking for a lawyer between the ages of thirty and thirty-five, with brown hair and blue eyes, who skis, plays tennis, loves cats, and is generally understanding and perfect in every way. Such people are often basically fearful of establishing a deep relationship with any one person, and they set these very rigid requirements (often unconsciously) in an attempt to exclude everyone. In this way, by blaming their plight on the fact that no one meets their standards, they avoid facing other emotional problems they have about commitment or self-esteem. This kind of pattern has caused some people to go on and on for years still looking for the ideal person.

It doesn't sound to me as if your daughter fits this category, however. Perhaps you and your husband are simply bothered by the fact that you were able to make your choice at a relatively young age and that your daughter is not. Keep in mind that life styles have changed and the goals that people have today are considerably different from what they were when you married. Don't pressure your daughter in any way or make her feel as if there is something wrong with her. Continue to communicate with her openly, and accept her individuality without forcing your own values and standards on her.

The Overindulgent Grandparent

What should parents do when grandparents spoil their children dreadfully? We have three children under nine years of age, and when they go to visit their grandparents, they're indulged in everything their little hearts desire. My husband and I are concerned that this sort of inconsistency in discipline will confuse our kids in the long run. Are we right to be concerned?

If you and your husband are each consistent in establishing the rules and regulations in your own home, and if your children have a deep sense of trust in each of you, it is highly unlikely that overindulgent grandparents will cause any psychological problems. If, however, these indulgences are conducted in a conspiratorial manner or are based on untruths (such as "Don't tell your parents about this—it will be our secret" or "It's silly that your parents won't let you do those things, so we will"), that's another and more harmful matter. It is clearly destructive to have your authority undermined in this way.

I see nothing wrong with saying to your children, "I know Grandma and Grandpa let you do most of the things you want—even things we disapprove of—and that's all right in their house, but it is not acceptable here at home." However, prepare yourselves for some manipulating statements, such as "If you won't let me do it, Grandma will." Your answer should be "That's something that you and Grandma can work out yourselves, but as far as I am concerned, I forbid it." Do try to communicate openly and show respect for your parents' feelings. If you find, however, that their indulgences are in fact causing a real problem among all of you, make it clear to them that you will be forced to consider restricting the children's visits. While no one likes to do something like this, remember that your primary responsibility is to your own children. They need the strengthening guidance that you, as parents, provide.

The Great-Grandparent as Babysitter

My grandmother is lively and sweet but quite elderly. She lives close by and often offers to babysit for our children, who are two and four. I'm a little fearful about leaving them with her—after all, she is quite old—but she seems hurt by my refusal. Is a woman of eighty-five able to cope with two small children? Should I allow her to do it?

I certainly think that you should allow her to help you in some way, because it benefits everyone. It is marvelous that your children have an opportunity to relate to an older person who is "lively and sweet." I am sure you greatly appreciate her help, and at the same time she must gain a great deal of pleasure from being important to you as well as to her two great-grand-children.

However, it is not totally unrealistic to have some reservations about whether she can cope with children of two and four. I don't care how old an adult is, children of this age can be awfully negativistic, defiant, and rebellious at times and can pose a threat to *anyone's* well-being. Perhaps it will give you more peace of mind if you leave your grandmother with the children only fairly short periods of time. You might also call her frequently while you are away simply to see how things are going. This would preserve the meaningful relationship you all have with each other—and diminish any anxiety you might have.

Retirement

My husband retired several months ago, and since then he's sunk into a real depression. He used to be outgoing, but now he just mopes around. What do you think is the matter?

In a study done at McGill University, my colleagues and I investigated the psychological and physical effects of retirement. We found that during the first six months after retirement it was very common for a period of turmoil and depression to set in.

Perhaps the best thing you can do is to encourage your husband to engage in activities that concern others. Some newly retired people become involved in projects with local schools, churches, and government; some enroll in classes or take the opportunity to travel; and some find special satisfaction in immersing themselves in family activities, particularly those involving grandchildren. Once your husband's life has become busy again and he has been reassured by friends and relatives around him that he still plays an important part in their lives, his depression should subside.

Widowed Older Parents

My widowed mother is seventy-five years old, and she seems to be constantly on the go—she's in church groups and exercise classes and making plans for travel. My brothers and sisters and I urge her to take it easy, but she just won't listen. Isn't it our responsibility to keep a woman of her age from exerting herself in this way?

Your widowed mother is to be admired for her energy, independence, enthusiasm, and vitality. It is highly unlikely that she is exerting herself beyond her limits. In fact, it is probable that her energy and enthusiasm come from the personal gratification she must get from being so active.

She sounds like a marvelous person, and I hope she continues to ignore your urgings to take it easy.

My father-in-law is in his middle fifties, and has been widowed for several years now. He has just announced his intention to marry a woman who is twenty-nine. She's a lovely person and they seem very happy together, but I must say our family is rather taken aback. Isn't there a problem when there's such an age difference between marriage partners?

The age difference need not be a problem. In fact, there are many marriages with this sort of wide age difference that have survived far longer than marriages in which the age difference was minimal.

Perhaps your family should reexamine their true feelings. You might discover that your own hesitancy in supporting this marriage is unconsciously based on selfish motives—concern over your inheritance or some threat to your existing family relationships.

When you really get down to it, this sounds like a wonderful event. I suggest that you share their happiness and give them full emotional support for their new life together.

Pregnancy and Your Feelings

As I approach my final months of pregnancy, I'm doing everything I can to be happy and relaxed—I play my favorite music often and garden, and when people ask me what I'm up to, I reply that I want the baby to be feeling nice things, and maybe be interested in them, too, someday. My husband, though, says an unborn baby doesn't respond to any of this. Is that true?

Old wives' tales to the contrary, there is no evidence that what you actually do during your pregnancy can influence what your child's interests ultimately may be. There are, however, sufficient data based on animal studies and even some human studies showing that extreme stress or unhappiness during pregnancy can have an effect on the offspring of the mother. Clearly, unborn babies are dependent on the functions and well-being of a mother's body—her nutritional condition, the drugs or medication that she may take, and her hormone balance (which *does* relate to the mother's emotional state). In much this way, if you feel relaxed, happy, and content, it can have an effect on your hormones, which can in turn have some effect on the child. What these effects are is not clearly understood, but I hasten to add that there can be no harm whatsoever in doing what you are doing; in all likelihood your pleasure and your relaxed state will make your pregnancy more enjoyable, and perhaps give you a better feeling about being a parent when your baby arrives.

Our baby was born prematurely and had to spend the first several weeks of his life in the hospital. Now that he is home with us, should he be treated with any special care and attention? Do premature babies have any emotional problems as their childhood progresses?

I am sure your doctors have given you advice about the physical care of your child. In respect to the baby's emotional health, it is not necessary for you to treat a premature baby with any more special care and attention than you would an infant born after a full-term pregnancy. I think it is essential to give your son as much cuddling, love, and stimulation as he requires. In this way he will develop a trusting relationship with you and will flourish emotionally. Babies who get a great deal of cuddling, both premature and full-term babies, seem to be more outgoing and friendly and more independent later on.

While there is no reason to think that premature babies will have any particular emotional problems as their childhood progresses, babies who undergo a great deal of stress and require a great deal of medical attention so early in their lives may show more difficulties with growth and development. In some instances, they may seem more sensitive to light or sound or show a greater degree of irritability in certain situations.

But perhaps the greatest stress lies in the forced separation of the parents from the newborn baby. I see what I consider to be a normal depression on the part of parents who are not able to touch their babies or hold them while they are in their incubator. While this separation need not be detrimental to your child's emotional health, a parent may have some perfectly normal feelings of deprivation at this time. For this reason, we at the New York Hospital—Cornell Medical Center encourage our parents, and some grandparents, to come to the special-care nursery where premature babies are housed, so that they can have physical contact by reaching in to touch their new babies. In fact, whenever possible we allow the parents to take the baby out of the incubator for small periods of time and even to begin breast feeding when the baby is physically able to handle it. It is a real delight to see the expressions on the faces of these parents when they hold and caress their tiny offspring.

Can Infants Smile

I eagerly reported to my mother that our four-month-old baby smiles happily at her father and me, and my mother said, "Oh, that's from gas." Is this really why infants smile?

No, that is not at all why infants smile. It is very common for babies to smile as early as the first week of life, and at this time the "smile" is a rudimentary reaction of the facial muscles, occuring at the end of a feeding when the sucking need has been gratified (this helps infants to detach themselves from the breast or the bottle as they relax and go off to sleep). Mothers and fathers then automatically smile back, and the stage is set for the development of "social smiling" later on. As weeks pass, the smiles of babies turn into positive emotional reactions to a warm parent-child relationship.

Do Infants Know the Difference?

Our four-month-old son is often left in the care of grandparents and other family members. I would like to know if a baby recognizes the difference between his parents and the others who pay so much attention to him. My aunt says that "everyone's the same to a baby," but I insist that our baby knows my husband and I are special.

By the time babies are four months old they certainly can differentiate between their parents and other people, provided those parents have spent a considerable amount of time with them. In fact, I am convinced that babies learn the difference between their own parents and others much earlier than this. Most parents have noted how a newborn infant, during the first days of its life, will look up into its mother's eyes during feeding. The baby begins to associate such gratifying experiences not only with the mother's face but with her smell, her taste, her touch, the sound of her voice, and the movement of her body. It is for this reason that I strongly advocate that both fathers and mothers spend considerable time with their newborn babies—in order to establish this bond.

There is nothing wrong with other people caring for the baby, provided they too have feelings of warmth and an understanding of the baby's needs; but I think it is important for the child's own parents to be the primary people in his or her life. Your aunt, though, would like to believe that "everyone is the same to a baby" and that *she* is as important to your baby as you are. I am sorry to say that many people such as your aunt may envy you for having your baby and may unconsciously show their envy by trying to take away some of your pleasure. I often wonder if people who continually undermine your confidence in such ways are not "repressed kidnappers," trying to carry off some of the joy that they wish they themselves had.

Breast Feeding and Weaning

Just how long should a mother continue to nurse a child? I'm still breast feeding my baby after sixteen months, and many of my friends say this isn't good. Is there any set time when nursing should be stopped?

There is no specific length of time that a child should be nursed. Some mothers do continue to breast feed longer than you have, but I think it is important that a child start achieving more self-sufficiency around two years of age, and it is wise to begin weaning him in other ways at least by that time.

My main concern about this point is that mothers not prolong breast feeding because of her own desire to keep their babies dependent on them. I have seen many babies give up breast feeding themselves because they seem to find it too confining—they apparently have less desire for the close physical contact they needed during the first year of life. My own son gave up breast feeding quite spontaneously at ten and a half months; it was as if his need was satisfied and he wanted to get on with other things. I do think that most children have had enough breast feeding by the time they are around eighteen months.

An important point to remember is that babies have a very strong need for sucking satisfaction during the first year of their life, and this need must be met in order for it to go away effectively. Since weaning a baby from a breast or bottle before it is eighteen months old usually intensifies its need for sucking for a longer period of time, I'd much rather prolong nursing or bottle-feeding and make sure the baby's need is satisfied instead of cutting off prematurely something the infant still instinctively wants to do.

Regardless of how long the baby nurses, most babies seem to cling to a need for a breast or a bottle at bedtime even beyond two years of age. While the daytime need may have been curtailed, the nighttime need will persist for a longer time—but this is both common and understandable.

I'm awaiting the birth of my third child and have had every intention to breat feed, as I've done with my other two children. My husband, though, wonders if it's a good idea for our five- and seven-year-olds to see me doing this.

What happened when your seven-year-old was two? He was probably more fascinated then than he will be now. As long as you treat breast feeding as a totally natural and tender process, and answer questions without embarrassment, the children will accept the whole thing.

I can easily understand this father's concern. My son was six years of age when he first observed his sister breast feeding. I was extremely curious to know his reaction as he observed the process with great intensity and wide eyes. "What do you think of it, Eric?" I asked. "Boy, is that neat!" he said.

My husband and I are expecting a new baby, and we'd like to know what explanation we should give our four-year-old about the physical process involved in the whole thing. How much should a child of this age be told?

A four-year-old's questions are usually a serious attempt to gain understanding of one of the great fascinating processes of life. The average four-year-old can be told the following: "A baby grows from an egg. The eggs are made in a part of the woman's body called the ovary; and one egg—it is a very tiny thing about the size of the head of a pin—goes from the ovary to the uterus [not "the tummy"] once a month. If the egg is fertilized by a seed from the man, it begins to grow in the uterus. It takes about nine months for the egg to become a full-grown baby."

I recommend that you have a book available containing pictures of a growing fetus so that you can explain to your child how the new baby is developing from time to time. You can explain the various stages, such as when it has little fingernails and when it is able to open and shut its eyes, and this will increase your child's fascination with the whole mystery of life. You can further explain that "when the baby is ready to be born, the woman goes to the hospital where the doctor helps the baby come out." This explanation will help the child anticipate and prepare for a separation experience when the mother eventually leaves for the hospital.

If the questions go on, particularly as the child grows older, the one that seems hardest for parents to handle is "How does the seed get from the father into the mother's uterus?" I find that children can easily accept the following explanation: "When two people love each other very much and decide to live together and have a baby, they often feel like hugging and kissing each other a lot. At times, they are so close and happy that they almost feel as if they want to be inside each other's bodies. When this happens, the man's penis is put into the woman's vagina and that's how the seed—which grows in a man's testicles—gets from the man into the woman. When this happens, it makes both the man and the woman feel very good, and this is something you will understand more about when you grow up."

You can expect that your child may ask, "The next time Daddy plants a seed in your vagina, can I watch?" Just explain that "this is something people like to do when they are alone."

I know that many parents are apprehensive about giving this type of explanation for fear that their children will tell other children around the neighborhood. If this is the case, you can say to your child, "Not all parents believe in telling children these things. It might be best if you don't explain it to your friends, but let their own parents explain it to them."

I feel quite strongly that children's questions concerning reproduction should be answered honestly, directly, and in a way that is understandable for them. Otherwise, children may pick up misinformation about the matter, or may see and hear things over the nine months that could be upsetting or even psychologically damaging if they have no idea what is really happening.

My eight-year-old made a very matter-of-fact comment about sex the other day, and when I asked him where he heard that he said, "From my friend's mother." My husband just laughed and said it didn't matter where our son got his information, but I'm not so sure. My husband and I have been rather evasive when our son asks us about sex, and now I wonder—is it harmful for children to pick up sexual information at random like this?

It is extremely important for parents to be honest with their children about all matters. Most children begin to wonder about sexual matters around the age of three or four, but their questions usually concern reproduction rather than sex. If parents answer those initial questions frankly and in a simple way that satisfies a child's curiosity, the child will be far better equipped to understand other sexual matters later on. If parents *avoid* answering such questions throughout the normal course of their children's growth and development, children will be vulnerable to confusing and even false ideas from other sources.

Parents who avoid the topic of sex are not protecting their children; in fact, uninformed youngsters are far more likely to get into trouble. After all, refusing to teach children how to cross busy thoroughfares doesn't prevent them from venturing out on their own one day and being hit by automobiles. It is not mere chance that our country's birth rate—which has dropped for mothers in all other age groups—has not decreased among teenagers, and many experts believe that a lack of basic sex education accounts for this.

Words to Describe Sex Organs and Body Functions

I was raised to use "cute" words for urination and genital organs, and a lot of little children I know still use words like "pee-pee" and other such babyisms. Now that my own child is two, I wonder what words I should be teaching him.

I see no harm whatsoever in using made-up or baby words if you feel more comfortable this way. However, you can avoid potential confusion for your child if right from the start you are as straightforward as possible. Why not call a penis a penis? Why not call a vagina a vagina? These words have no negative connotations, and there is no need to avoid their use. I do understand, however, that the use of specific terms can be awkward in some instances. For examply, the term "urinate" seems rather clinical and long compared to the word "pee" or "pee-pee," especially for a two-year-old who is grappling with the new use of language. Similarily, it may be a little too much to expect a two- or three-year-old to use the word "defecate." But a term like "bowel movement" or "BM" is descriptive, direct, and less clinical or complicated. As I said, I see no harm in using any term with which you are comfortable, but it might be easier and less confusing in the long run if the terminology relates more directly to the function you are describing and at the same time is easy for a child to say.

Parental Nudity in Front of Children

My husband and I occasionally walk between bathroom and bedroom without our clothes on. Our two children, ages four and six, don't seem to notice this particularly as yet, but friends say that our behavior may have an adverse effect on them sexually. We want our children to develop open, healthy attitudes toward their bodies. What are your feelings about nudity in the home?

I think that the casual attitude you and your husband have is a healthy one. Being natural and matter-of-fact about nudity prevents your children from developing an attitude of shame or disgust about the human body. If parents are very secretive about their bodies and go to great lengths to prevent their children from ever seeing a buttock or breast, children will wonder what is so unusual and even alarming about human nudity. More often than not, such secrecy intensifies a child's desire to know about what is being so explicitly hidden from view, and it can cause distorted ideas about nakedness and sexuality later on.

Incidentally, children themselves may eventually go through periods when they are very modest about their bodies and may not want anyone to see *them* naked, even their own parents. The phases sometimes take on rather amusing variations. I remember when my little daughter developed a great feeling of modesty about anyone's seeing her navel—a concern that seemed strange, since she had no qualms whatsoever about exposing the rest of her body. Phases such as this come and go—and during them parents should do their best to respect a child's privacy.

You've obviously handled the situation well if your two children see nothing strange in your casualness about nudity. By being open, honest, and direct in dealing with matters such as this, you contribute to your children's emotional stability—much more so than if you try to withhold imformation and act as if the natural elements of life are mysterious and forbidden.

(I must add that I am not advocating that parents go to the opposite extreme and parade around constantly in the nude, or lounge about in erotic poses. Nudity in this form *can* be sexually provocative and confusing to a child.)

Parental Privacy During Sex

A friend told me her child walked in while she and her husband were making love. It made me wonder what I would do if my five-year-old son appeared in our bedroom at that particular moment. How should we handle it?

Most people, when this occurs, react as if they were doing something wrong and have been caught at it. They should not act this way. But it is important for you to show your indignation and dissatisfaction over his intrusion on your privacy, without becoming irate and terrifying him.

Shortly after the interruption has taken place, it is also important to explain to the child—who may be frightened and think his mother and father have been hurting each other—how much the parents love each other. Explain to him that sometimes when you kiss and hold someone whom you love, you become very excited and want to be very close, almost a part of the other person's body.

As far as privacy and sex are concerned, a paradox arises becauses many parents ordinarily allow children free run of the house, including the bedroom. I think it is important to establish some rules of privacy that can be applied at *all* times, so that children realize they cannot simply barge into the place to which someone else has gone in order to be alone.

Sex and Birth Control

When my nineteen-year-old daughter came home from college for the holidays, I inadvertently discovered that she was using birth-control pills. I'm quite upset and don't know whether to confront her with this information. What should a mother do if she finds out her daughter is engaging in premarital sex?

If you are quite upset about finding that your daughter is taking birth-control pills, you should bring up the subject with her; otherwise, your feelings of discomfort will come out in some irrational way.

If you have had an open and understanding relationship with your daughter, matters of reproduction and sex have been discussed easily between you. This closeness would set the stage for a frank discussion that would reduce your discomfort now.

I am sure, however, that nothing she says will put you at ease completely. It is important to remember that the average parent of a nineteen-year-old grew up at a time when birth-control pills were not available and premarital sex was definitely frowned upon. However, times have changed tremendously. There is now a greater openness about contraceptive methods, and premarital sex is more acceptable today than ever before. Your daughter cannot help responding to the customs of her era rather than to those of yours. I know that this thought does not make it easier for parents, but they must recognize the fact that times have changed, whether they like it or not.

Do no hesitate to express your feelings about these matters to your daughter. Whether she agrees with you or not, it is advisable for you to explain—in a manner that is not dictatorial or disapproving—the emotional implications and possible consequences of what she is doing. Make it clear that she should always feel free to talk to you about any matters that trouble her. But understand that your daughter is at an age of independence and operating within a different set of mores and attitudes from those that prevailed during a similar stage in your life.

Vulgar Language

Both of my children were polite, friendly, and well-behaved until they started going to school. I find now they're picking up ugly words and expressions, which they use openly in front of my husband and myself. Should we do something about this, or is it just a stage?

In all likelihood they are picking up these words and expressions from the children with whom they go to school. During play-period, lunch time, and going to and from school children mingle more freely with each other than they do in the classroom. Teachers generally have more control over the environment at that time. At these other times, some children who want to bully others, intimidate others, or generally arouse a startled reaction, demonstrate behavior patterns and language which is frequently socially unacceptable. Understandably, other children, such as your own, who are exposed to this, find themselves doing the same thing. If you think back to your own childhood you'll remember hearing words you hadn't learned at home which, to be sure, your parents would have been horrified hearing.

I recall, when I was seven, my best friend Billy, who lived next door, asking his mother how to spell a very specific four-letter word he had heard at school. I was somewhat shocked at the casualness with which his mother responded. She went on to explain that some people try to be "big shots" by using these words and think they are upsetting people when they do. She simply pointed out that nobody particularly enjoys hearing these words and simply added that you would probably lose more friends than you would gain if these words became part of your vocabulary. Billy had a very trusting relationship with his mother—she was what I consider to be "an askable parent." That means that Billy was able to check with her when it came to understanding things that confused him, or were simply mildly perplexing. If she had taken a very strong punitive stand and absolutely forbidden him to use these words ever, in all likelihood he wouldn't come to her with his questions, nor would he be able to learn her feelings about this language and the possible consequences of having these words become part of his vocabulary.

There is no way you can control the language your child uses in all situations. If you take a very punitive or extreme stand on an issue like this, you may intensify your child's fascination with these words and make them more important than they really are. I believe you can handle the situation best by letting him know that you just don't like hearing these words and expressions and have no intention of carrying on conversations when these words are used. Point out further that you know that people you respect feel similarly. Don't hesitate to point out that the "shock effect" of these words is what causes some people to use them extensively. Don't hesitate to tell your child that people who are unhappy inside themselves tend to need such words and expressions as devices for getting people to react to them, whereas people who are stronger and happier within themselves don't need to use them.

Bathroom Humor

In the middle of conversations—with anyone, on any occasion—my six-year-old son will suddenly announce that everyone is doing "doo-doo" in their pants, and laughs uproariously. Even though he obviously thinks this sort of "bathroom humor" is the height of hilarity, I wonder if I should be doing more to squelch it. Or is this a stage all youngsters go through?

Your six-year-old is going through a normal stage. Children around this age are often somewhat crude in their social interactions, and they simply roll with laughter when discussing any bathroom activity. As a parent, you should guide your child and at the same time show acceptance of his feelings. You can tactfully take your son aside and explain, "I can understand that you think this is terribly funny, but not everyone does—some people don't like it when you say things like that." In this way you are acknowledging your child's feelings about what he considers amusing but at the same time offering guidance by explaining other people's reactions to this behavior. If you allow your son to go through this normal stage in development and set the limits and the circumstances under which his "jokes" are permissible, you will find that his interest in "bathroom humor" will diminish with time.

Masturbating

From time to time I find my five-year-old engrossed in playing with his penis. I don't want to make him think there's anything shameful about doing this, but I'd like to make it clear that he can't stand around doing it in front of people either. How should a parent react to this?

I think your attitude is a very reasonable one. You recognize the fact that he is going through an exploratory experience that is perfectly natural and you are right to be concerned that he not develop a deep sense of guilt about this. Nevertheless, you are also right in thinking that it is not the sort of activity that a child should be engaging in publicly.

Take a matter-of-fact approach, indicating that you understand the child's impulse to do this. At the same time, explain, "If this is what you want to do, do it when you are alone and not when there are others around." Don't be harsh or punitive in your attitude. Try to communicate the fact there's nothing wrong with a child's touching himself in this way, but it is not an activity others enjoy watching.

Children go through stages when they engage in more masturbatory activity than they do at other times, but generally speaking they will not do it escessively unless there is a significant emotional problem or they are living in a somewhat unstimulating environment. Some children engage in greater masturbatory activity if the parents are overly strict and force them, as a form of punishment, to be alone in their rooms without anything to do.

Playing Doctor

A few days ago I came upon my six-year-old daughter and several of her little friends—boys and girls—pulling down their underpants and examining each other. Should I fuss, or forget it?

Generally speaking, the activity that these children are involved in is perfectly normal and represents an almost universal curiosity that is usually satisfied by playing "I'll show you mine and you show me yours."

I don't think you should overreact to the "game" by expressing strong disapproval or by taking punitive measures; your overreactions may intensify the child's feeling about sexual exploration, and that intensity may in turn lead to increased sexual activity or to the complete suppression of healthy sexual desires. Nor do I think you should ignore the activity—it is important for children to realize that they are doing something that is not socially acceptable. And finally, I certainly don't think you should merely sit by and watch because it's "cute."

What you *should* do, in an offhand way, is let the children know that you've seen them playing a game you think is sort of silly. Suggest to them that they play something else. By giving this game a mildly forbidding aura, you can make clear that bottoms and genitals are not to be examined casually and at the same time impart the idea that sexual stimulation and pleasure have a special significance.

Don't be surprised if in spite of your urging this

happens again—it's perfectly understandable for a child to be fascinated by his or her own body and the bodies of others.

Sex-Role Identification

From a very early stage in her life my three-year-old daughter has insisted she is a boy and refuses to wear dresses or frilly things. In games she assumes the masculine role, and prefers to play with toys associated with boys. Should I insist she wear dresses and try to talk her out of her attitude, or permit her the fantasy and let her dress and behave as she pleases?

I have seen this kind of thing occur very frequently in little children, much to the horror of their parents—and the more horror parents express, the more the pattern of behavior is reinforced.

I do not think that this situation necessarily reflects an emotional problem; instead, it probably indicates your daughter's tendency to identify with the role of the father, the male. Generally speaking, this phenomenon occurs as a result of environmental experiences in which the child sees the male role as the more satisfying. In many instances, children who show this behavior pattern simply change it spontaneously sometime during childhood or puberty. In any event, I do not think that you should insist that she wear dresses or try to talk her out of her attitude. If you do, you will simply be increasing the intensity of her desire—out of stubborness—to take on a male role, which would probably irritate you even more.

I would like to add this general comment: I think it is important for us to downplay the importance of sex-role stereotypes to our children. The responsibilities and interests of the parents should be interchangeable enough in every way so that a child does not make a sharp distinction between the mother role and the father role.

We have three very feminine daughters (ages five, seven, and nine) and a two-year-old son who loves them and spends most of his time playing with them. My husband and I wonder if he'll suffer any hangups by being exposed to three extremely feminine girls on this developmental stage of his life. And should we be doing anything to help him develop his own male identity?

There is no reason whatsoever to fear that he will suffer any hangups as a result of his family constellation *as long as* he has a good, solid, meaningful relationship with one or both of his parents, based on *his* individuality. His identity as a person, as well as his identity as a male, will emerge spontaneously if his individuality is nurtured in this way. While the pleasure he gains from playing with his "feminine" sisters may lead him to engage in the kind of play they do, generally characterized as having a feminine quality, most children show periodic fluctuations in the kind of interests they have. Boys playing with dolls is nothing to fear, any more than girls playing with cars, in my way of thinking. The more children's play departs from sex-role stereotypes, the easier it will be later on for them to share in the roles and activities they will engage in as parents.

Pornographic Material Around the House

My husband sometimes buys those glossy, soft-core pornographic magazines and is very casual about leaving them around the house. Now that our children are getting older—our son is three and our daughter is almost five—I'm concerned about their seeing the photographs in these magazines. My husband says they're "not old enough to be bothered." Is he right?

Children of this age, and for that matter any age, are generally very curious about all sorts of things. It would not surprise me at all if they do notice these magazines, However, taking notice does not necessarily mean that they are "bothered by what they see." In fact, even at a later age their curiosity about the pictures in these magazines may still not really "bother" them. It is perfectly possible that your children will show little or no interest after their initial curiosity is satisfied.

Generally speaking, most people, children included, eventually become bored by this kind of literature. But if parents act as though it is taboo and impose severe restrictions and penalties concerning it, they are making the issue more important than it really is—and adding a "forbidden" dimension that makes the whole thing exciting to a child. It also must perplex children, who wonder what it is that makes you so upset over something that seems relatively uninteresting. If the situation is as casual and as "soft-core" as you state, and if the children see that you regard nudity in a healthy and matter-of-fact way, I don't think these magazines will cause any emotional disturbances.

The Pacifier

My two-and-a-half-year-old still sucks a pacifier day and night. We have tried to ignore this habit in the hope he would give it up on his own, but so far he hasn't. What should we do? And what is your feeling about pacifiers?

Let me begin by telling you that I do not like the use of pacificers in the first place. I think it far better that babies have a sensation of something entering their stomach while satisfying their sucking need. In this way, the child associates the sucking gratification with the intake of food. If a pacifier is used, it becomes an end in itself. Moreover, during early infancy many parents give a baby a pacifier every time he cries. But oftentimes babies cry because they need cuddling and play, and using a pacifier in this way means the baby is plugged up rather than picked up. If this happens, your baby may be receiving less of the cuddling and sensory stimulation that is so important for healthy emotional development. In addition, the sucking response may become a substitute for any other kind of satisfaction that a child needs when feeling uncomfortable. I feel that sucking should be gratified —but in a functional way, with the intake of food.

Now that your two-and-a-half-year-old is dependent upon this pacifier, it will be somewhat of a disappointment to him to have to give it up. If he still takes a bottle, I think you should simply take the pacifier away and let him have the bottle at the times when he wants the pacificer. If your child is no longer on the bottle, tell him that he can "have it today and tomorrow and the next day—and then no more." Each succeeding day remind him that in a short time he will no longer be having it. But this preparation does not mean the pacifier will be given up willingly when the time comes. You can be almost certain that he will be somewhat upset and angry when he finally learns that what you have told him is true. At that time it is important not to return the pacifier but to offer him additional cuddling and comforting.

Oral Satisfaction

My four-year-old son puts everything he comes across directly into his mouth. I've locked up prescription drugs and dangerous household chemicals, but it is impossible to keep everything out of his way. What can I do to protect him from hurting himself? Is it normal for him to be doing this?

It's unusual for a four-year-old to put *everything* he comes across into his mouth. It's common for children between birth and two years of age to do this. I certainly think you have taken the best precautions possible by keeping dangerous things out of his reach, but I do believe it's possible to talk to a four-year-old about the possible hazards involved in doing what he is doing. If he ignores you or still compulsively puts everything in his mouth, then I believe you should seek professional help.

In my experience, babies who were weaned too early, or were not allowed to satisfy their sucking needs during the first few years of life exhibit a tendency like your four-year-old's. In a sense he is trying to seek satisfaction now for his unfulfilled infantile needs. Parents who are quick to wean their children or deprive them of satisfaction for their sucking needs in a comfortable and gratifying way frequently find that this frustration can lead to a preoccupation with oral behavior. During infancy it's appropriate for a baby to find satisfaction and pleasure in sucking at the breast or bottle. Unfortunately many people feel the need to stop this satisfaction for fear that it will cause a child to want continuous oral stimulation. It's quite the opposite, as you have found out. The best way to make a need go away is to satisfy it as the need arises. This is certainly the case when it comes to eating. If you avoid eating when you are hungry, it simply intensifies your hunger and interferes with all functioning, including the way you see the world. People whose hunger is satisfied find that they can devote their energies, both physical and psychological, to the tasks at hand.

Attempts by parents to force a child to give up what is biologically necessary at any given stage in development accomplish quite the opposite. This problem you are having with your four-year-old is far easier to prevent than it is to treat.

Thumb Sucking

My three-year-old sucks her thumb, and no matter how many times I gently pull it from her mouth and say no, she puts it right back in again. Why is she doing this? What should I do?

During infancy a baby has a strong need for sucking gratification, and if this need has been frustrated—as a result of a rigid feeding schedule or because the baby was not given sufficient sucking time during feedings—a child may continue to need to suck a thumb or some other object. This will be most likely to occur when children are tired or under emotional stress. As time goes by, their thumb sucking gradually diminishes.

Nevertheless, thumb sucking can persist even if a child is emotionally secure simply because the behavior has become a mindless habit. It is not harmful in itself, but it can be bothersome to many parents. Parents are usually exhorted by relatives and friends to "do something about it," and they resort to punitive methods, such as painting the thumb with bitter substances or severely punishing the child. But this sort of reaction can hurt the child far more than the thumb sucking. The only dangers of prolonged thumb sucking might be deformities in the formation of the child's teeth, but in my experience these deformities are more readily correctable than are the emotional scars that can result from harsh or humiliating punishment.

Most children give up thumb sucking spontaneously when they get to nursery school and kindergarten simply because they are embarrassed by the reaction of their peers. But even though this kind of embarrassment generally does the trick, I am totally aginst *parents'* ridiculing the child for the same thing. I see no harm, though, in gently hinting that she should remove her thumb from her mouth. Do it in a casual way—if the child gets the idea that you dislike the habit so much, she may suck her thumb simply to gain negative attention.

Be patient and provide your child with sufficient love and stimulation, particularly at those times when stresses in her life cause her to turn to her friendly thumb for security and gratification.

Stuttering

For the past several months my six-year-old son has been stuttering, which upsets him terribly—and upsets us as well. At times when he's trying to say something, he gets so frustrated by his stutters that he starts to cry. Am I wrong to hope he'll grow out of this? Or is there anything at all I should be doing to help him? He's a very bright child, and my husband and I have a very good relationship with him. What could be causing this?

Stuttering is often a transitory phenomenon that occurs when a child is under undue pressure or has experienced some frightening event. When the pressures are diminished or after the traumatic event has passed, the stuttering ceases spontaneously. Many children who have never stuttered or stammered before do so when they begin school for the first time or when a vacation is over and they are adjusting to a new teacher or a new class situation.

It is indeed frustrating to a child who wants to say something and can't get it out. The best way to handle this situation is to be extremely patient and avoid getting upset yourself. Your son must sense the fact that the stuttering worries you and your husband, and this simply serves as an additional pressure on him. You cannot force a child to stop stuttering or punish or ridicule him out of it. When parents handle a problem this way, it simply gets worse and sometimes causes a child to avoid communicating altogether. Instead, since periodic stuttering is a barometer of the amount of emotional pressure a child is experiencing, try to reduce the pressures on your son as much as possible. Give him the opportunity to express all his feelings, and give him your unconditional support when he does.

If stuttering persists regardless, it may be necessary to look for some underlying emotional problem. In general, a child's inability to communicate represents some fear that he will say something unacceptable that might cause his parents to reject him. If a child has repressed certain hostile and aggressive feelings—and fears that they may come to the surface—stuttering and stammering may be the result. If your child's stuttering persists even after you have done what you can to allay his stress, you should seek professional psychological help.

Lisping and Infantile Speech

Our five-year-old daughter, who talked very plainly and well at age two, has now begun to talk with a lisp, like a baby. We have asked her why she's doing this, and she's said she just wants to be a baby again. Is this behavior natural?

It is not natural for a five-year-old to "just want to be a baby again"—unless a new baby has arrived in the home and the older child has been substantially neglected as a result. The fact that she turns to "baby talk" indicates some unfulfilled need. Your daughter obviously feels that being a five-year-old does not provide her with the kind of emotional gratification she needs, and you should make special efforts to give your child some individual and undivided attention.

Speech problems frequently begin at the age of five, when children go off to school for the first time. Their regressive speech patterns may mean that they do not like their new-found independence and they may need extra loving assurance and encouragement at this time. Do not, however, intellectualize the problem and try to discuss with her the irrationality of her behavior—you will get nowhere, as you have already found out. But you should discourage her infantile speech by making it clear that you do not care to communicate when she speaks in this way and asking her to speak more clearly and more properly before you respond. Do not make a big issue of this, but simply, without preaching, reinforce her positive behavior and ignore the negative pattern.

Exposure to Foreign Languages

I'm part of a warm and close-knit family, and since many of the members are second- and even first-generation Americans, my new baby often hears a language other than English. What kind of influence does this have on a baby's early speech development? Should I curtail the family visits?

I would certainly not curtail the visits of your relatives—if they are warm and loving, the security and happiness they give your baby is far more important than the language they speak.

Early speech development is basically influenced by the one or two adults whom the baby is around and whom he trusts the most (in this case, as in most cases, his parents), and the influence of other relatives and friends is really incidental. It is best, however, not actually to teach such a young child more than one language, because the child may mix words from the two languages and end up with a limited vocabularly in both. As a general rule, a small child should learn one language well —and later, at the age of two and a half to three and a half, can begin to learn a second language often spoken in his presence.

Physical Differences in Appearance

We have just learned that our thirteen-year-old daughter needs to have glasses. She refuses to wear them, though! How can we convince her otherwise?

It is extremely difficult, if not impossible, to force a teenager into anything without causing some loss of face for someone—either parents or teenager. Remember that this is an age when young people are deeply concerned about peer pressures and are attempting to exert their independence and individuality. Ironically, in their efforts to show their individuality by doing precisely what their parents do not want them to do, they generally show extreme conformity in doing what their peers do.

I'm sure that the more you press this issue, the more she will resist. In fact, it is possible that her absolute refusal to wear glasses stems directly from your insistence that she do so. By simply explaining to her the consequences of not having this optical correction (or even better, the positive reasons *for* having it) and by pointing out that the problem really is hers and not yours, you may be opening up the lines of communication between you. If your daughter feels that she has various choices in the matter, it will enable her to assert herself and at the same time make a choice that is in her own best interest. You might ask her if any of her friends wear glasses, and offer to give her free rein in picking out whatever frames she likes. As an additional possibility, you can mention contact lenses. In any event, the most important thing is to respect her wishes, offer her options, and help her solve this problem for *herself*. Most teenagers, when presented with this sort of situation, will make their choices in a sensible manner.

My granddaughter—she's now eighteen months—was born with a very noticeable birthmark that extends down the entire side of her face, and we've been told nothing can be done about it. We now wonder how best to protect her from the questions and comments of the other children as she grows up.

Clearly, this can be a stress situation for a child, and it is all the more reason that emotional stability should be established during the child's early life. In fact, children who have been taught at a young age to cope with their frustrations and anxieties are much more capable of dealing with the stresses that life offers later on.

I don't think you can protect a child completely from the questions and comments of other children, but you can certainly help prepare her for dealing with them. When your granddaughter asks about the birthmark, you should convey the idea that all people are different in some way—by saying, for example, "Some need to wear glasses and some don't, some people are tall and others short. Others may even be deaf, or unable to see. You were born with a birthmark, and it was nothing that anyone could help; just as many people learn to live with many different things, you must learn to live with this."

The child should be told that some children may tease her about the birthmark, but many people will just look at it in a curious way when they first meet her. Explain that after people get to know her they probably won't even notice it.

The important thing is to be open and to encourage the child to talk about the matter honestly with you. In this way, you will be helping her to learn to deal with the stress of having this minor defect and to develop her own resources to deal with the situation.

Toilet Training

I have a twenty-four-month-old son who is being toilet-trained. The woman at his day-care center never has any problem with him about using his potty seat, and when my husband is with him he has no problem either. But when I'm with him, he goes to the bathroom in his playsuit or pants. I swear he does it on purpose every time! Is it possible he has a problem with me? How should I deal with it?

Clearly he reacts differently to you than he does to the other significant people in his life. I'm not sure I would classify this as a problem, but I would certainly say that somewhere in his behavior is a message for you. Although he has relinquished an infantile pattern in relating to his father and the women at his day-care center, he is telling *you* that he still wants to be a little baby. Perhaps he feels more secure in his relationship with you when you treat him in this way.

Many children are not fully toilet-trained until they are closer to the age of three, and I feel this is a more realistic age toward which parents should aim. Moreover, children under the age of three still require a great deal of parental time and attention; they are not quite ready to cope with long periods of time away from their parents without showing some resentment. If you have been the primary person in your son's life, it would seem logical that he express this resentment and the need to remain close to his family—to you.

At this point, I don't think you should make a drastic change in his life situation, but perhaps you ought to give him more undivided time and attention and shorten his time at the day-care center. I should add that, as a general rule, I do not advise people to put their children in day-care centers but to try to work out an arrangement where both parents can participate in caring for their children at home—perhaps with the assistance of a part-time baby-sitter.

If you satisfy your child's craving for time and attention during this stage in his development, he should then be able to resolve his infantile needs and will not carry them on into adult life, where they may reappear as neurotic symptoms that emerge to provide partial satisfaction for needs never met in childhood.

For months now my four-year-old son has been holding back his bowel movements. He can go for as long as four or five days, until we're forced to give him an enema (which he resents very much). My husband and I have become very upset about this, and we wonder if there is some psychological reason for his behavior. And if so, is there anything we can do about it?

It is absolutely essential for your child to have a careful medical checkup to see if there is a physical cause for this. But even if the problem is psychological—and most often it is—I feel it still should be managed with the help of an understanding and patient pediatrician.

Sometime between twelve months and three years of life, most children develop the idea that their bowel movements are literally part of their bodies. During this time it is normal for children to show concern about parting with their feces—they may show a reluctance to have it flushed down the toilet or may even wave "bye-bye" as it goes down the drain. Other children may become terrified if someone flushes the toilet while they are sitting on it, fearing that some important part of themselves is about to be lost forever. Or a child may actually get stuck in or slip through a toilet seat, and the experience may frighten him badly. Any or all of these associations could cause a child to "protect" himself by holding back his bowel movements. Also, during toilet training a child may have learned that his parents regard his bowel movements with significance. By withholding them, a child may be trying to preserve something that he has learned is important.

Enemas are frightening to children (and many adults, too!). They will probably intensify your child's fears and add credence to any idea he may have that you are trying to take something away from him or are determined to control his bodily processes. Unless he is quite seriously impacted, it would be best to speak to your pediatrician about a laxative to help things along. This, together with your patience and understanding, should make it possible for him finally to overcome his fears.

I have had a number of cases like this during the past years, and they are indeed difficult for both child and parent. In some instances, further counseling or psychotherapy was needed when parental patience and a laxative were not enough.

Bed Wetting

My older children—they are ten and fourteen—are bed wetters. It's a habit that embarrasses them and annoys me, and I just don't know what to do. Should children of these ages still be having this problem? Should I try to shame them out of it?

No, children of their ages should not be wetting their beds, although it is not really that unusual. And no, you should *not* try to shame them out of it. This sort of tactic never works and can cause severe emotional upset and feelings of rejection that will only intensify the problem.

Bed wetting can be caused by a number of factors. It could be due to environmental pressure and tension and, if so, will subside when the pressures are removed. Sometimes it is due to emotional problems within the child, which will require some professional psychotherapeutic help. In most instances, though, I think it is due to some organic factor, and it is often associated with children who are high-strung and have a tendency toward hyperactivity.

In any event, I think you should consult your

pediatrician about this so he can check for physical causes and discuss with you your children's emotional state and any stressful situations that might be taking place in your home. Some pediatricians recommend medications that help children stay dry through the night. Other doctors may recommend electronic devices that wake children up as soon as they wet, but I am absolutely opposed to these. I have treated some adult patients in psychotherapy who developed worse symptoms as a result of using these machines.

I think the best approach to the problem is to have your children place a loud alarm clock some distance from their beds and set it to wake them three or four hours after they go to sleep. After getting out of bed to turn off the alarm, they can make the trip to the bathroom. The alarm clock should be reset for the same time interval throughout the night. The children can set the alarm for a longer and longer time interval, and ultimately they will overcome the problem. This method gives the children a sense of mastery over their problems.

Accident Proneness

Our five-year-old son is always hurting himself. It seems he can't walk across a room without spraining an ankle or cracking his skull open on the corner of a table. None of our other children seem so accident-prone. What's going on?

Accident proneness in children this age can be the result of awkwardness caused by poor muscle coordination. In most instances this changes with time as a child's muscle coordination improves. However, some children who have frequent accidents like this may have a neurological disorder or a form of epilepsy which causes them to lose consciousness momentarily. Other neurological disorders can cause a child to simply collapse but regain muscle control in a matter of seconds. This is not a problem to be diagnosed by parents themselves, but the symptoms of frequent accidents or falling should be a warning sign that your child needs to be seen by a pediatric neurologist.

In some instances accident proneness is caused by emotional factors. When a person harbors a great deal of hostility and anger, or feels caught in a double bind, or if he is damned if he does or damned if he doesn't some form of aggression turned against himself results. In a sense it's a way of venting pent-up emotions that can't be resolved in any more direct manner. While this kind of disorder is not frequent in children, the symptoms warrant medical attention. Even if you suspect that the problem is caused by emotional factors, it is still wise to investigate the possibility that some nervous-system disorder is causing poor coordination or occasional lapses of consciousness.

Problems of the Short Child

My child is quite small and seems to have trouble keeping up with her age group. I know she is a bit immature and I am sure she will grow up soon enough, but right now I am worried that she doesn't have enough friends. Should I leave well enough alone?

No, I don't think you should leave well enough alone. Frankly, things are not well, since your daughter is having trouble keeping up and lacks sufficient friends. I also think that your being worried is also a good reason to consider doing something about the problem. Parents—aside from the occasional overprotector or superworrier—frequently have good instincts about problems. Under the best of circumstances raising children is indeed a tremendous responsibility, with all its normal everyday problems. Adding more anxiety than is necessary to this responsibility serves no one's best interests.

Children who are small in stature suffer a lot—particularly among peers who are competitive. Along with feeling inadequate, they sometimes get to feel resentful and angry and take out their resentment on children even smaller than themselves. They also become more vigilant about their strengths and weaknesses, which can lead to more despair later on.

Perhaps you ought to reevaluate the situation with an eye toward having your daughter associate with young people more within her "size" group as well as at her level of social maturity. While I'm generally not in favor of having a child repeat a grade for these reasons, it is sometimes the best arrangement, since it places a child in a more appropriate group with respect to size and social maturity. The problem becomes one of handling such a transition diplomatically and in a way that does not give the child a sense of failure. Here is where your ingenuity in conjunction with the diplomacy of a school can go a long way. In my experience this can sometimes be worked out best by having a child move to another school.

Seeing the Dentist

I know it's time that our six-year-old should be seeing a dentist, but a neighborhood child told her the dentist is "scary" and would hurt her. Now she's so frightened that whenever I mention the subject, she cries and carries on! How do you prepare a child for her first visit to the dentist, especially after she has already been frightened?

A trusting relationship with a dentist or doctor is basic to the development of proper health habits. Just as your child's trust in you enables you to offer her emotional security and protection in matters of everyday life, so will your daughter's trust in her doctor and dentist encourage her to take advantage of the best in medical and dental care.

Tell your daughter that her friend is not being fair when she describes the dentist this way. You can even talk about the fact that it's your daughter's friend who's really scaring her, and not the dentist at all. Then I think you should have a frank discussion with your daughter about dental care in general. Explain that if people eat the proper foods and take good care of their teeth by brushing them regularly, dental problems will be less likely to occur. Explain also that regular visits to a dentist often keep problems from developing. In this way you are reassuring her that dental care, for the most part, prevents pain rather than causes it.

Suggest to your daughter in a friendly, casual way that the two of you visit the dentist in his or her office, simply to say hello and see what kind of a place it is. Then, when an actual examination is scheduled, it will be by someone your daughter knows and not a totally unfamiliar person. Don't hesitate to contact your dentist to get assistance in preparing for your child's first visit. He or she is likely to have helpful literature on this subject provided by the American Dental Association. And if you feel the dentist does not react with understanding about this sort of situation, then ask other parents to recommend a dentist who does. This way you can give your daughter the proper introduction to good dental care and set up positive habits and attitudes that should serve her throughout her life.

Facing Doctors and Hospitals

My seven-year-old has to go to the hospital for an operation, and her grandmother keeps telling her that "nothing's going to hurt." Is it right to mislead a child this way?

It is specifically this kind of situation that causes many children to lose trust in adults. A child is sure to find out rather quickly—especially in this sort of instance—that she has not been told the truth, and she may then begin to disbelieve almost anything adults say. Oftentimes such children later become discipline problems; they refuse to cooperate with grownups who have offered them no real support in upsetting situations—and who have also misled them and left them vulnerable to pain.

It is far more honest and respectful to the child to tell her the truth—that "something is going to hurt or be uncomfortable for a little while, but it's because everyone wants to help you—and we'll understand if you feel like crying." By doing this, you give your daughter the encouragement to mobilize her own resources to cope with an unpleasant situation.

She may now brace herself and come through it all without hysterics or tears, in which case you can say, "My, how brave you are—I know it hurt and you didn't even cry." On the other hand, if the child does cry, the adult can say, "Yes, I understand—it does hurt." Either way, the child has had the opportunity of using her own abilities to deal with a real situation, and has the compassionate backup of an adult.

My friend took her two-year-old child to the hospital for surgery and left her there all night. Later, my friend found out that another mother had stayed with her child all night "with her doctor's permission." What is the best thing for a parent to do in cases like this? Are children ever psychologically damaged by such experiences?

When overnight hospitalization is necessary, it is definitely better for a parent to stay—particularly when the child is very young. If a child is older and indicates a desire to be alone, clearly that is another matter. However, hospitalization is generally very frightening, and I have seen many problems resulting from a hospital experience where the parents did not offer enough comfort to the child.

Most hospital procedures obviously defy a child's wishes, and most young children interpret all this as a hostile experience that the parents could have prevented had they wished. The fact is that young children in this situation are often resistant and fearful, and they deserve all the support and parental attention possible.

Unfortunately, many parents are regarded as "overanxious" by hospital personnel when they are simply showing what I consider to be appropriate anxiety and a normal protective feeling toward an ill child. Also unfortunately, in the past some children have shown disturbed behavior patterns following even a brief hospitalization. They later have been suspicious of doctors and nurses, many of them have had problems sleeping, and many tend to cling to their parents and show a great deal of emotional insecurity. On the other hand, I have seen many children who have come out of the hospital with a minimal amount of psychological discomfort—because they were prepared for surgery by a medical and nursing staff who gave the children an honest and sensitive description of what they would be experiencing. I am happy to say that more and more hospitals—with the help of organizations such as the Association for Child Care in Hospitals and the Society of Pediatric Psychology—are doing their best to protect children's integrity and self-esteem by offering their compassionate reassurance at this difficult time.

Refusing to Take Medicine

Our fourteen-month-old son has a minor infection, and the doctor prescribed medication that he must take orally. But my son firmly resists, and I often end up forcing the spoon into his mouth. I feel terrible. Am I hurting him psychologically?

I certainly can understand your feelings. It is very common for youngsters to dislike taking medicine, and parents feel awful if they must force a child to do so. I would suggest that you give your son his medication as quickly and painlessly as possible, then offer comfort immediately afterward.

I have often wondered why pediatricians do not provide parents with a disposable syringe (without the needle, of course) into which the medication could be drawn. The syringe could then be placed into the child's mouth more easily than a spoon, which often ends up being tipped in the scuffle and makes the situation more disorganized than it need be.

It is highly unlikely that episodes such as this will have any long-lasting psychological effect—especially if you and your child have a good relationship to begin with. Unfortunately, when children are this age, getting medication into them is no easy task and often does require force. The only reasonable antidote to this force is understanding, love, and tenderness when the incident is over.

Explaining a Nervous Breakdown

My children, who are ages eight through thirteen, love their aunt—my sister—who lives in a nearby town. But recently the problems in my sister's life have built up and she has had a nervous breakdown. I've simply said that "Aunt Fran will be away for a little while," but I know she'll be coming home soon and the children will want to see her. How should I explain the situation to them? Or should I just avoid the subject, and keep the kids away for a while?

If you avoid telling your children about their aunt, you miss an opportunity for teaching them about some of the realities of life and their resolution. Also, they may later resent you for having kept the matter a secret and wonder why you didn't consider them worthy of sharing this information. I can certainly understand your desire to protect them, but I think it's far more important for you to be honest with them and at the same time help them cope with their feelings about their aunt's difficulties.

Explain to your children that their aunt had many problems that caused her to be very tired, upset, and overwhelmed. (And don't underestimate the sensitivity of your children in understanding what these feelings are like—even in their young lives they know.) Tell them that when the pressure becomes too great, it's necessary for some people to back away from things for a time, to rest and think before finally getting back to their normal life again. Explain that this feeling of being so absolutely overwhelmed is often called "a nervous breakdown" and that sometimes people go to a hospital so that they can be in a quiet place where all their needs are taken care of and where people are on hand to help them feel better. This, incidentally, is an excellent opportunity to tell your children about psychologists, psychiatrists, social workers, and other health professionals.

The fact that your children want to visit their aunt confirms that she is important to them and that they love her. Perhaps you should let your sister know this, since it will be very reassuring for her to know that everyone misses her and is eager to see her again. I think, however, you should wait until your sister actually returns home to see how she feels about having visitors. And if she feels she *doesn't* want to see people for a while, make it clear to your children that this is not a rejection of them but simply a way of making it easier for Aunt Fran to adjust to being home again.

They say my child is hyperactive. I am trying to give him some extra activities after school, but most children won't play with him because they say he's too rough. What can I do?

Hyperactive children frequently experience feelings of rejection by peers and not infrequently by their own parents. In general, they have trouble sitting still in school and focusing their attention and are often so impulse-ridden that they speak out of turn or run out of class. They have difficulty learning because of this inability to focus their attention for a sustained period of time.

In my experience as a psychologist, I have consulted with parents, teachers, and children concerning hyperactivity, its causes, and treatment. In the large majority of cases I have found that the symptom of hyperactivity has been caused by some neurological dysfunction. Also in the majority of these cases the children have been above average in intelligence and frequently emotionally strong, with the exception of some of the psychological problems their symptom of hyperactivity has caused. I've found that their major problem seems related to their nervous system's inability to shut out all the unimportant or extraneous stimulation that most of us seem able to shut out automatically, and so their capacity to think and focus attention cannot operate effectively in spite of the fact that their intelligence is normal.

A very large number of these young people, in my experience, have benefited enormously from the careful diagnosis of the problem and medically well-monitored use of medication that serves to activate that part of the nervous system—the inhibitory apparatus—which had not been functioning effectively enough to allow a child to be able to function well in social situations. Needless to say, this not only eliminates the problems for everyone, the child particularly, but it gives a child a sense of self-esteem which he would not otherwise have because of the tendency to reject him on the basis of his hyperactivity.

I believe you should have your child carefully evaluated by an experienced and competent pediatric neurologist and clinical child psychologist. With the help of a detailed developmental history—including the history of the pregnancy, the birth, and the immediate postpartum period, in conjunction with the neurological examination and specific psychological tests—in all likelihood a treatment plan can be worked out to help your child.

Not all cases of hyperactivity are due to neurological dysfunction. In some instances, it's a symptom related to anxiety and has more of a psychological than a physiological cause. In any event, the kind of evaluation I have suggested will serve to determine the likely basis for your child's symptoms, and if it is determined that it's due more to psychological factors than physiological factors, the appropriate recommendations can be made by the professionals involved in the diagnosis of the problem.

Understanding Aging Relatives

My mother-in-law, who has lived with us for ten years, is beginning to get senile at age seventy-five. This confuses our children—six and eight years old—very much. How do you explain to children what is happening to their beloved grandmother without frightening them?

Explain that Grandma has gotten to be very, very old and that sometimes when people get to be very, very old they have trouble thinking and sometimes find it very hard to remember. Explain that in some situations they even forget the names of the people they love and sometimes do not even recognize them. Let your children know that not everyone who gets old gets this way, but that it seems as if their grandma, who loves them very much, is changing. Make it clear that all the love she had for them in the past is still there, even though she cannot express it in the same way.

Point out to them that in no way did this happen to Grandma because of anything they did. Encourage them to ask you questions and do your best to explain things in a way that they understand. If you encourage a free-wheeling discussion about Grandma and the aging process itself, your children will be better prepared for one of life's most important realities. Show your understanding for their confusion and unhappiness about the changes in Grandma, but again, reassure them that her love for them was always sincere and will continue to be there, whether she expresses it or not.

Despite the fact that your children will be saddened by contact with their grandmother, I believe you should encourage them in it. It would not only offer comfort to Grandma but would also be a statement on your part of the importance of people regardless of how old they become or how ill they become. This is a message all young people should hear to enable them to grow up with respect for every stage in a human being's life. While it may be depressing for your children, offer them your support and pride in the expression of their continuing love for their grandmother.

Explaining Death

My husband is seriously ill, and the doctors tell us he can't be expected to live longer than six months. Should the rest of our family know this? Our children are six, ten, and thirteen, and I just don't know what I should say to them.

I think it is important for the children to know that their father is seriously ill; trying to "protect" them from this news, which they must ultimately face, would be both dishonest and impossible. But it is also important to sustain some feeling of hope. Explain that although the doctors do not expect their father to live for a long time, no one knows for sure how long he actually will live.

I also think you must do everything you can to maintain an atmosphere of openness so that everyone feels free to discuss and express his feelings. Let your children know that it is understandable for them to feel fear and great sadness. At times they may wish to share these feelings with one another; at other times, they may want to go off and cry by themselves.

It is true that some people urge everyone to smile through times of great hardship and show "bravery." This attitude only causes one to foster tremendous feelings of guilt and weakness. It is right and natural that human beings experience grief and sadness in this kind of situation. It should be made clear to your children that tears are not synonymous with weakness but are instead an appropriate expression of deep feeling.

My seven-year-old daughter was very close to her grandmother, and when her grandmother died last month we were quite gentle about breaking the news to her, thinking she would take it very hard. But our daughter seemed to accept the news quite matter-of-factly, and although she talks about her grandmother from time to time, she doesn't seem to be showing any particular grief at her death. Is it natural for a child to be so unaffected by the death of a loved one?

I am sure your daughter *is* deeply affected, even though she does not show the kind of grief reaction that you expect. For the most part, children began to show their greatest reactions to the death of a loved one when events continue to take place in everyday life and that loved one is no longer available to participate in them. This kind of grief reaction often predominates during various holidays and other family events such as weddings, anniversaries, and birthdays.

The fact that your daughter is able to speak openly about her grandmother is a very good sign. It means that her grandmother still exists in her mind and that the child is relating to her in this way. Seven-year-old children often engage in fantasies that to them are almost the same as real experiences and that give them a great sense of fulfillment. Perhaps your daughter is still engaging in many activities with her grandmother—not in the real world but through the marvelous fantasy mechanisms that take place in her mind.

I would encourage you to talk openly with your

daughter about her grandmother and feel free to describe your own feelings—let her know that you miss Grandmother and feel fearful and grief-stricken at times. But it is not necessary for your daughter to have precisely the same feelings or reactions you do.

My elderly father lives close by and my family sees him often. Lately, he's been making more and more references to how we're going to miss him when he's "gone," and he talks about friends who have "passed on." But he seems in good health, and I find his remarks quite unsettling. What should we all say when he talks like this?

Obviously, your elderly father is worried about death. This is understandable, because it becomes more of a reality as time goes on. He is also reacting to the grief that he feels as he loses his own close friends. He is also probably wondering how important he really is to you, and whether you will in fact miss him when he is gone. When he makes a comment about his death, you might say, "Father, I know you are worried about death. We all love you very much—you have always been an important part of our lives and will continue to be so, whether you are here or you are gone. Of course, we would miss you a great deal if you weren't here." You might add jokingly, "The more you talk about it, the more upsetting it is—you're in such good health that you'll probably outlive us all."

Ever since our family cocker spaniel died, our four-year-old daughter has been asking where it is and when it's coming back. How should we explain to her what death is? Or should we just get another dog quickly and postpone any explanation until she's older?

It would have been best to deal with your daughter's problem at the time your dog died. In fact, it would have helped matters a great deal if she could have participated in some form of funeral ceremony and burial. Not only would it have answered the questions concerning the animal's whereabouts, but it would have been an appropriate time for the expression of sorrow over the loss of a close and loyal friend.

With all good intentions, many parents want to protect their children from the reality of death. But the death of a pet offers a natural opportunity for helping a child come to terms with something that sooner or later will have to be faced.

I know it is difficult to explain an abstract concept like death in concrete terms, but it is important to do so. A four-year-old will want to know specific things, such as why a person or pet can no longer do the things he used to do and why parents and doctors can't do anything about it. The death of your dog should be explained as "like being broken and no one can fix things again—not even the doctor." You should add "this can happen because of a serious accident or sickness—or when you are very, very old." This will be more comprehensible to a child between two and five than if he were told, "God took your dog away and he is in heaven." Then you are sure to be faced with such questions as "How did God take him away?" and "Where is God? Will He give my dog back to me?"

It is *not* right to tell your child that death is like

being asleep for a long, long time. This explanation may easily result in a fear of going to sleep.

After you have explained the death of your cocker spaniel to your four-year-old daughter, she may want to have another pet. But she should make that decision with your help and certainly with the understanding that she will still remember and miss her old friend.

I came home from school (I'm eleven and a boy) and found out that a lizard I had been keeping in my terrarium had died—and my mom had flushed it down the toilet while I was gone. I really liked that lizard very much and even felt like crying—I at least would have liked to bury it out in the yard—but I didn't say anything. Was my mom right to do that?

It's understandable that when you lose a friend or something or someone that you are close to, it makes you very sad. It is perfectly natural and right to express your unhappiness; there is nothing wrong with crying, particularly in circumstances such as this.

It would have been nice if you could have buried your lizard in the yard and even placed a marker on its grave. In this way you could have shown respect for your lost friend, and the "ceremony" would have helped you acknowledge and deal with your grief. After all, funerals and other such rituals that people engage in are for this purpose: to say farewell to a friend and, in doing so, attempt to come to terms with the sadness of a real loss.

I certainly think you should talk to your mother about this and let her know exactly what is bothering you. I am sure that she had no idea how deeply hurt you were, and you need to help her understand how important this was to you. Explain to your mother that in the future you want to handle matters like this in your own way. If it has been your responsibility to care for a pet when it is alive, you certainly should have the opportunity of making final funeral arrangements after it has died.

It is important for family members to talk to one another about how they feel, and if you keep all this to yourself, your mother will never have the chance to comfort you and be close to you. Lizards may not be important to parents, but their children's *feelings* about lizards are.

When an old family acquaintance died recently, we stopped at the funeral parlor to pay our respects and took our four-year-old inside with us. Later a friend told me how horrified she was to see us there—she said that the experience would have a morbid effect on a child. Do you think this is true?

I think it is important for children to recognize the importance of life by acknowledging people's reactions to death. While it is very difficult to accept the fact that all things ultimately die, a child feels more secure knowing that "loved ones" are grief-stricken, sad, and depressed when death takes place. "Paying respects" at a funeral parlor exemplifies the reality of death, and while this may be somewhat upsetting to children, it also provides an opportunity for helping them come to terms with this reality.

It is highly unlikely that a visit to a funeral parlor under normal circumstances will have a morbid effect on the average child. Sometimes actually seeing a dead person is upsetting, but more often than not, it is an experience mixed with curiosity and fascination. Such a visit will definitely precipitate questions. I recall one child asking, "Do you weigh as much dead as when you're still alive?" and "What happens to people's houses and clothes after they die?"

As a general rule, I believe that people should be honest in answering children's questions concerning death. These questions should be answered in a literal and concrete way until children are approximately five years of age, after which time it is possible to offer explanations that may have some religious or supernatural significance. In my experience, children under the age of five have a great deal of difficulty understanding explanations such as "God took Grandpa away because he wanted him." Little children then may become very angry with God, and in one instance a child announced that when he grew up he was going to *find* God and tell him he wanted his grandpa back. It is far better to give young children an explanation like the one I suggested before—that death is "like being broken, and no one can fix you, not even a doctor or nurse."

Sleeping with Parents

My four-year-old loves to crawl into bed with her daddy and me, and up to a point we love to snuggle with her, too. But this frequently happens at all hours of the night, and when we try to turn her away she cries dreadfully. Should young children be allowed to sleep in their parents' bed, and if not, how do you stop them?

Understandably, children get to enjoy being in their parents' bed and cuddling up to protective adults—it makes for that lovely feeling that all is well and nothing can go wrong. As a general rule, though, young children should not be allowed to sleep in their parents' bed. It can cause a child to develop an unhealthy dependency on the parents, as well as drastically infringe on the adults' privacy—and many psychoanalysts are adamant in their recommendation that this *never* happen. I cannot take such a hard line as that, however. There are some extenuating circumstances, and if a frightened or uncomfortable child occasionally crawls into bed with her drowsy parents and is left there until morning, it will not be damaging to anyone involved.

It is important, though, that this not become a regular habit, a habit that is much easier to prevent than it is to cure. It is best to explain to children that they have their own beds and really should sleep there. When a child comes into your bed at night, it is possible to offer the reassurance that he or she is seeking by taking the child back to his own bed, perhaps lying down with the child and explaining that "I will stay with you until you go to sleep and then I will return to my own bed." There may be protests and tears, but I think it is far better to help the child learn to cope with the situation himself, in his own room and bed, rather than give in to the problem and find later on that a pattern has been established that not only undermines the child's capacity to master occasional nighttime fears but also interferes with the privacy of the marital relationship.

Winning and Losing

Whenever I participate in any sort of simple game or sport with my children (ages four and six), I play fair and square. If I win, I say so, no matter how much tearful sulking is done by the losers. When visiting grandparents play, however, they tell our children, "You win, you win," whether they did or not. I get annoyed by this. Should I be?

I can understand your concern, but it really isn't worth getting upset about. You probably feel that the grandparents are spoiling the children by doing this. They aren't. Your children will catch on, if they haven't already, that this is their grandparents' way of pleasing them and of getting special affection in return.

I agree that children have to learn to accept defeat as well as success, and they certainly should be dealt with honestly. On this issue, the grandparents aren't being exactly honest, and I think you have the right to discuss it with them, explaining that the children will respect them more in the long run if they play fair.

I must add, however, that I don't think grandparents should have to conform to all of the parents' values and ideas—as long as they do not undermine the parents' authority. In situations where grandparents are clearly overindulgent, you can tell a child that "even though Grandma and Grandpa give you whatever you ask for, it doesn't change the rules in our house." Even a young child can understand the difference in these relationships (this is also a good way of teaching youngsters that grownups are "people" too), and the child should feel more secure because you have maintained the discipline and values he or she is familiar with.

Recently I took my eight-year-old son and my seven-year-old daughter to a local fair. Sarah proudly won a stuffed toy and, although David played more and more games trying to win something, he was unable to do so—and was miserable for the rest of the day. How should a parent handle such a situation?

Children whose reactions to winning or losing are very intense and prolonged are usually responding to their underlying feelings of insecurity or to parents who have placed undue emphasis on competitiveness and winning. I don't mean to imply that anyone who enjoys winning is insecure or has overbearing parents, but I do feel that if the desire to win or the discomfort of losing detracts from the pleasure of participating in a game or activity in the first place, then things are not as they should be.

In your case, your daughter's pride and your son's dissatisfaction sound like no more than transitory and understandable emotional reactions. The best way for you to handle the situation you describe would have been to acknowledge your children's feelings. You might have said, "Sarah, you must be very proud of yourself for having won!" and assured David that, while he must have been a little disappointed, you were proud of him for having tried as hard as he did. By taking a casual attitude about this but at the same time acknowledging your children's feelings, you will let them know that you understand and sympathize with their reactions, but at the same time your love and acceptance of them has nothing whatsoever to do with their success or failure at games.

Every time we take a picture of our son he insists on taking the camera away so that he can take a picture, too. Unfortunately, our camera is a major investment and we were very upset when he took a picture and jammed the shutter. How can we teach him to respect other people's property?

One of the major ways children learn is by imitation. When your child sees you taking pictures, particularly with a camera that you value so greatly, he, too, wants to get involved with this object. Your taking pictures is, in a sense, "play activity," as he sees it, and, understandably, he wants to have fun playing with you. Any attempt on your part to keep him out of the "game" would indeed be frustrating and unfair. His resentment and anger could cause him to become destructive and feel rejected by you.

Obviously, you have to draw the line somewhere when it comes to a child's desire to imitate everything you do. Driving the family car is not by any means an activity that I recommend for eight-year-olds simply because they want to learn. However, I think occasionally using the family camera to take a picture is justifiable, *but* you must let your child know what the rules are and how to do it. I'm sure he didn't deliberately jam the shutter in your camera, and in no way can I interpret this as disrespect for your property. I suggest that on occasion you let him take a picture but show him precisely what to do and how to do it. If photography is among your major interests, you might consider getting your son a camera of his own that is simple and inexpensive yet gives him the opportunity of participating in an activity similar to that of his parents. By giving your son a camera, you encourage his individuality and show respect for his curiosity and desire to share in his parents' interests. At the same time this will give you the opportunity to see his work product, which can lead to a greater sense of self-esteem for your child.

Photography happens to be one of my own personal interests, and my daughter, when she was nine years of age, was given a camera that was easy to operate. I was absolutely fascinated by the things she photographed and her ingenuity in picking subjects that were meaningful to her. After learning from some of her mistakes concerning the use of light and distance, she had fewer and fewer failures and was ultimately able to use the camera to demonstrate her talents as a photographer. Needless to say, she was able to share her accomplishments with her friends and teacher at school, not to mention the adulation she received from me because of the great pictures she took. It would never have occurred to me to photograph pebbles through clear, shallow lake water, but it did her. Her photographs of flowers, clouds, and even insects tell me a little bit more about the world in which I live as seen through the eyes of a young person. To me, this is a great gift that children can offer the adult world.

Allowances

My eleven-year-old says that all her friends have allowances and begs to have money of her own. What do you think about allowances? Should they be given at all—and if so, what amount?

I think children should be given allowances to help them develop feelings of responsibility and independence about money. I do not believe that parents should withhold a child's allowance as punishment, nor do I feel that it should be increased for "good behavior." It should be a fixed amount that is given the child regardless of the circumstances. If you withhold it as punishment or increase it as a reward, this will intensify any association a child may make between the acquisition of money and feelings of emotional security or love.

It is impossible for me to recommend a specific amount of allowance, since that should be determined largely by the parents' economic situation and by the general standards of the community in which you live. I suggest that you use your own economic standards as a guideline. Some parents are inclined to overindulge their children by giving them large allowances to compensate for the lack of time they spend with them. If you live in a community where this happens, it can create an unfortunate situation: your child, aware that a friend gets a larger allowance, may feel somewhat deprived. If this is so, you have to explain your own position clearly and firmly.

Hoarding Money

While other kids are squandering money on comic books and candy, our twelve-year-old son hoards his allowance, keeping track of every penny and even charging other children interest on any money they borrow from him! At first we thought his tightwad tactics were amusing, but lately we feel his obsession with money has gone too far. Should we be alarmed that our son feels this way? We want him to handle money thoughtfully, but we don't want him to be miserly or attach undue importance to it. How do we do this?

Frankly speaking, your son's behavior is extreme. While I don't think you should be alarmed about it, it's important for you to try to make inroads into his current view of money. Encourage a more flexible attitude about money and let him know that he should use some of his money for his own pleasure and perhaps share these pleasures with his friends. If his sole pleasure seems to come from hoarding, he is, indeed, showing miserly behavior. Let him know that charging interest on loans to his friends is hardly a friendly gesture and can cause him to be looked upon as strange, or perhaps even to be rejected by them.

Strange as it may seem, your son's hoarding and miserly attitude about money can have its origins in the way he was toilet-trained. When toilet training is coercive and conducted in a manner where the parent places a great deal of value on the child's feces, children sometimes hold back on their parents. In a sense, hoarding it and then discharging it gives them a sense of pleasant relief from any discomfort, while at the same time they are trying to retain something that their parents have placed a great deal of value on. If a child is offered parental acceptance when he does the right amount in the right place at the right time, and in the right way, and if they show a strong punitive attitude when the child does what he wants when he wants in the amount that he wants and the place that he wants, his feces have become currency for interacting with his parents and give him a sense of power in controlling them. When this association is made, it often manifests itself in the unconscious mind in conjunction with money. Holding back money is similar to holding back his bodily products, which give him control. It is precisely this control that he wanted but couldn't have, since his parents coerced him in a punitive way into giving them what they wanted and in a way they wanted it.

With greater parental understanding of the meaning of toilet training to a child, it's possible to prevent behavior patterns such as this one, or perhaps an obsessive concern for neatness and cleanliness, which sometimes grows out of confusion that takes place during the toilet-training process.

Cooking Together

My seven-year old son loves to cook and I like to encourage him in his interests. But how do I teach him that cooking can be a dangerous pastime and that he simply must have me around to supervise?

Let him know how pleased you are about his interest in cooking and also let him know how much you love him and care for him. Point out that because of this you don't want to risk anything happening to him and that you have to set certain rules about his cooking. Explain to him that rules are necessary no matter what you do, that they apply to all games and all activities. Perhaps you can start by explaining what he can do on his own to show him the wide range of freedom you will give him, and then let him know specifically what it is you don't want to do at the present time to avoid his causing harm to himself. For example, you might point out that he can use the electric mixer and can measure out the ingredients, which he can then put in a pan, but that he is not allowed to light the oven without your being there. Let him know that, as time goes on, and as he gains more experience, you will use your judgment to give him more and more freedom to do the things he wants. Emphasize the fact that you are not restricting his freedom but are simply protecting him from some possible dangers.

You are not alone with your problem. In fact, there are a few delightful books written with your specific problem in mind, which might be helpful to you in conveying to your son that cooking can be fun as a joint venture without any hazards.

Protecting the Family Pet

Our family cat is taking a beating. The kids in our house squeeze her and swing her and bundle her into doll carriages. My husband says the animal is fine and not to worry about it, but isn't it important to teach your children to treat their pets nicely?

Yes, it is important to teach children respect for animals—and for people as well. But children are inclined to be egocentric—or, more plainly put, somewhat selfish: they expect the cat to share their own playful feelings about what they are doing.

Sometimes children who have pent-up anger direct it at pets and can be rather cruel. If this occurs, it should be a message to you that your child has emotions that need release, and you should find out more about the anger or frustration he is venting. In this case, however, it seems to be a matter of your children's playfulness rather than malicious intent. But regardless of the intent, pets sometimes do need your protection and, if a game seems to be getting out of hand, you can intervene on the pet's behalf—and take that opportunity to explain that animals have feelings, too.

Delegating Parental Responsibility to Others

We have a live-in housekeeper who takes care of our four preadolescent children. Often they refuse to obey us and defer to her. Other times they are rude to her and will only listen to us. How can I resolve this peculiar problem?

Frankly, this is not a peculiar problem. It's very common in families where the housekeeper is delegated the responsibility for taking care of children when the parents are not there. The person you delegate this responsibility to psychologically represents *you.* Whatever resentment your children may have about her they can easily displace onto you and vice versa. This seems to be partly what has happened in your case. There is no way parents can hire someone to take care of their children and have that person offer the same emotional experience and the same values and elicit the same responses.

It's frequently very confusing for children to have someone in a position of authority as a parent surrogate who is not a parent. By the same token, children wonder how important they are in the lives of their parents if their parents delegate parental responsibility to other people.

I don't mean to sound critical of this arrangement, yet there is no way I can consider it the ideal for raising children. It has its problems, as you have found out. When you have two authorities who disagree or, at best, are not always in tune with each other, you can expect your children to react to the discrepancies.

Perhaps the best approach to your particular problem is to set standards concerning rudeness and make it clear that you will not tolerate their speaking to or reacting to *anyone* in a rude manner, and that includes your housekeeper. I would not set standards for her that are different from those for others.

On the issue of their refusal to obey you, it's important to keep in mind the fact that all children at times show defiance and rebelliousness. This defiance and rebelliousness may be assertiveness, which is part of the process of establishing independence and showing their individuality. If, however, it is an expression of defiance based on resentment for having to be with someone else in authority, then your approach would have to be different. In this case, explain to your children that you know they are not happy having someone else tell them what to do, but, unfortunately, this is the way things must be. If you let them know that you understand their plight and recognize their wish to have more regularity in their lives, they at least will understand that you are sensitive enough to their feelings but have to deal with the practicalities of everyday life in a way that makes it impossible for you to run a home without the help of a housekeeper.

All children want to feel important in the lives of their parents whether or not their parents work, have housekeepers, or travel. As long as your child knows and feels that he or she comes first and is deeply important to you, these problems will be minimal.

Talking to Strangers

Now that our children—they're six and eight—are venturing outside our home and becoming more and more independent, I feel it's necessary to prepare them for problems they may encounter. But how do you warn children not to talk to strangers without inhibiting or alarming them?

For some strange reason, parents think that simply telling children not to talk to strangers will prevent them from getting into trouble, but actually it is a blanket rule that is sure to inhibit and alarm them. Moreover, this kind of flat statement doesn't really help them understand or learn to deal with unpleasant situations that may occur.

I think it is best to tell children that there are some unhappy people in the world who are "sort of like sick people" and have become that way because of unfortunate experiences in their lives. You should indicate that they are not necessarily dangerous people, although on some rare occasions they do harmful things to other people. You can explain that sometimes they seem friendly to children and may even offer them candy or a ride in a car, or even suggest that a child come home with them. Point out that it is unwise to accept any of these offers unless they know the person very well. Make it clear that if your children abide by this rule, there is almost no chance that any harm will come to them in their experiences with other people.

You may want to mention other things that children sometimes encounter, such as persons opening their clothes to show themselves naked or grownups who try to touch the children's genitals. Put these in the same context of strange adult behavior that is "like being sick." and tell them they are right to be frightened by it.

In other words, it is important that the children understand the specific circumstances that might lead to danger—and how to cope with them if they occur. Suggest that if your children see or are pursued by such a grownup, they immediately find some other adult and ask for help. You can also encourage your children to talk to you about such incidents that my alarm them—this way the children need never fear that they too will be thought "bad" if they report an unpleasant happening. By handling the problem in this way, you are preparing them for some of the realities of life, offering a concrete way to deal with these problems, and not creating alarm or inhibitions about dealing with other people.

I have a four-year-old daughter with a real gift of gab. She has yet to meet her first "stranger," since she considers everyone from the mailman to the checkout clerk in the store to be her personal friend. She will soon be walking to school alone, and I'd like to know how to stress the importance of not talking to strangers without inhibiting her easygoing ability to strike up a conversation with anyone about anything. What warnings do you give a child of this age?

It would be a shame to spoil the trust of such a friendly child. Nevertheless, it is important for you to help her to cope more realistically with some of the hazards of everyday life. You can explain that there are some people who are "sort of sick" but whose illnessess "are not in their body but in the way they think and do things." Most children will then want to know "why people are like that." You can explain that people are not born that way but sometimes, because of the things that happen to them in life, they become upset and do strange things that are hard to understand.

You can mention some of the things you are specifically concerned about, such as her taking candy (or any food, for that matter) from someone she does not know. You can advise her never to get into a car or go off with someone who is unfamiliar to her. Tell her that if someone tries to force her to go somewhere, she should ask the nearest grownup to help her. Reassure her that things like this do not happen very often—you simply want her to know how to deal with these events if they do occur. In this way, you will be offering her techniques for coping with potentially upsetting experiences and at the same time reassuring her that most people are trustworthy and kind.

Bedtime Hours

I have always been a strict parent and have made my children keep lights out and bedtime hours, except for very special occasions. Now they're getting older—nine and eleven—and they have more energy than I do. Should I be more lenient?

Parents should always be flexible and should adapt their rules and regulations to fit the changing needs of their children. Moreover, I think it's important to take into consideration how the parents of their friends deal with similar situations. While I don't believe you should let other people determine how you run your own life at home, I do believe it's important for you to recognize the possibility that your children may feel the restrictions on them are far more strict than those of their friends. This can cause them to rebel against you and perhaps show intense open defiance of the rules and regulations you set up.

While I recommend leniency, I don't mean be inconsistent. When you alter the rules and regulations, let them know that you are doing it and why you are doing it. If you simply vary the limits you set without any explanation and do it in a very arbitrary manner, your children can become confused and anxious. I'm a firm believer in setting rules and regulations that are adhered to consistently, but I also believe in flexibility, compassion, and compromise. These are human qualities, and it's important for parents to demonstrate how and when to use them. When parents are compassionate and lenient and compromising, children respect them far more than when they rigidly adhere to rules and regulations that were set up for the "children's sake" and which cause them extreme frustration and even social embarrassment among their peers.

Postholiday Letdown

I dread my daughter's birthday. Each year she gets so excited and overwrought and inevitably she is disappointed by the end of the day. How can I deal with this yearly dilemma?

The disappointment children feel after an exciting event such as a birthday celebration is understandable. After all, no one likes to see an exciting event come to an end after a tremendous buildup. But, it's a reality of life that events like this come to an end and with the end comes the disappointment that it's over. The same happens during the Christmas holiday season, when families celebrate in their own way according to their own religious beliefs. The focus is generally on children, and there is great anticipation for the moment when they open their gifts and the surprise is over. The buildup results because children are frequently asked what they want in the way of gifts, and their fantasies and wishes are stimulated and given free reign. Not only that, but the ordinary rules and regulations or discipline of everyday life seem to be put aside during birthdays and these other holiday celebrations. Most of the "no-no's" concerning candy, cake, and other sweets, as well as bedtime and other restrictions, are generally put aside. The end of the birthday or holiday is the equivalent of saying, "Now we have to return to the real world and all of its limits, frustrations, and responsibilities. If every day were a holiday, the excitement of these special occasions would lose its spark." Although most parents point this out to children to help them with their disappointment, it generally goes over their heads. Most young people would prefer to live the world of Alice in Wonderland who proposed the idea of "unbirthdays" to enable us to celebrate 364 days a year what, in the real world, takes place only once a year. Alice's make-believe world may provide much satisfaction and happiness for children in their fantasies but in all likelihood would be a nightmare for most parents if it became a reality.

Watching Too Much Television

My kids—they're five through twelve—make an awful fuss if I try to curtail their many hours of television viewing. Is too much TV bad for them?

Yes, too much television is bad for a child—and for that matter, too much of anything is bad for anybody.

I must say that I think that many children are inadvertently forced into bad TV habits by their parents. When a parent wants some time alone or has been overburdened by a curious and enthusiastic child, it is too easy to say, "Why don't you go and watch TV for a while?" Some parents offer extended viewing hours as a reward, others take it away as punishment. And so the importance of television is enhanced.

I do feel, however, that television has some fascinating programs to offer, but as with all other forms of entertainment, it is necessary for a parent to provide guidelines. I think that a parent should help a child select programs that are emotionally and intellectually stimulating and then be firm in limiting viewing to these. It is also far easier to divert a child with an interesting book or hobby than it is to turn off the TV and offer no alternative at all.

It also should be mentioned that if children see adults watching indiscriminately for hours, it is hard for them to see why they cannot do the same.

Coping with the Brutally Honest Child

My three-year-old daughter is bright and articulate and has lots of friends in her neighborhood. Often, when they come by, she bluntly says she doesn't feel like playing with them; and on other occasions she'll send them home in the middle of a game. Her friends seem to accept all this, and I realize that children are brutally honest—but is there a way to "civilize" her a bit?

In evaluating a situation like this, it is always important for adults to look at the world through the eyes of the children involved. From the point of view of a three-year-old, her conduct is not antisocial but a perfectly reasonable response to her mood of the moment. I'm sure that her friends are, at times, as frank and abrupt as she is. As you yourself say, they seem to accept her behavior quite matter-of-factly.

I would say that there is no real problem at this time, but as a responsive parent, you recognize that if her behavior continues, there will be problems later on. On some occasion when you and your daughter are having a relaxed and happy moment together, talk with her about the possible consequences of her behavior. In a way that is not punitive or embarrassing to her, explain that it is important to be honest with people and to let them know how you feel, but at the same time it is important to think of how she herself would feel in the same situation. This conversation should make her more sensitive to the fact that her actions can cause other people to feel happy or unhappy. In a manner that is respectful and understanding, explain to her that if you make people uncomfortable by what you say or do, eventually they will not want to be with you.

Your comments, coupled with disappointments that may come to her later on because of her "brutal honesty," will go a long way toward encouraging what we adults call civilized behavior.

Christmas Syndrome

Every Christmas my children, five and seven, concoct elaborate lists of all the presents they want—and every Christmas morning, after they've plowed through all the nice gifts under the tree, they invariably say, "Isn't there anything else?" This always upsets me. Are they exceptionally greedy children, or do many youngsters act this way?

For children—and for adults, too, for that matter—Christmas time is very exciting and filled with many stimulating experiences. After all, children usually get to eat more candy, go to more parties, stay up later, and receive more presents than they do during the rest of the year. The wish that all this will "never end" prompts children to ask for more—they want the flow of gifts to be perpetual and they say so with the candid honesty that children are known to show. Some parents are upset when a child's wishes for "more" are voiced, but they should keep in mind that the momentum of the holiday spirit is at work and should deal with the situation by saying simply, "That's all there is—no more until next year."

Choosing Your Child's Playmates

We heartily disagree with the methods being used to bring up the young children next door: they're either subjected to swatting and screaming or ignored altogether. We feel that the bad effects of this sort of child raising may in turn rub off on our youngsters. Am I right to discourage the children from becoming playmates?

Undoubtedly your neighbors' children will show the effects of their parents' behavior, but this need not have any negative influence on your children. In fact, their friendship might give you an opportunity to offer the neighbors' children a greater feeling of stability and support and at the same time allow you to set an example for your own children in dealing with someone else's problems. If, however, the unhappiness of these children manifests itself in antisocial and destructive behavior, you can express your dissatisfaction and make clear to your own children the consequences of behavior similarly.

As a general rule, it is unwise to interfere with your children's choice of playmates. A child's reaction may be one of two extremes: he either accepts your choices, waits for your approval, and never asserts himself independently in relationships with others; or he rebels, secretly plays with those you discourage, and develops a resentment toward you.

In the end, it's best simply to help your children cope in their relationships with others. They must learn to make their own choices, and your role is to provide guidance and a lot of support when problems are encountered.

Tickling and Tossing

My husband plays with our two-year-old by tickling her and tossing her in the air, and I'm not always convinced that her screams are joyous. Is it possible to be too rough with a little child? My husband says I'm being overprotective.

It is perfectly possible for a two-year-old child to be overstimulated by this kind of activity. One would have to judge by her emotional reaction to what is going on. Often children will giggle with glee and all of a sudden show signs of fretfulness and anxiety. It is important for parents to engage in physical activity with their children that ranges from cuddling to friendly juggling, but it is equally important for the parents to be sensitive to the child's emotional reactions. In short, it is possible to be "too rough" and it is also possible to be overprotective. The ultimate judgment depends upon your daughter's reaction, and only her parents have the sensitivity to make this judgment. If you are in conflict over her reactions, perhaps each of you can compromise a little. Your husband can be less enthusiastic in his play, and you can be less prohibitive in what he is doing.

Messiness

My kids range in age from twelve to seventeen, and I think that the way they dress and wear their hair is terribly sloppy. But my criticisms don't seem to do any good. How can I get them to take more interest in their appearance?

Adolescents often rebel against parental values in order to establish their own sense of independence. Your comments about their appearance probably convince them all the more that they are accomplishing their purpose—they know you notice and disapprove.

I don't think that it is at all harmful for you to express your feelings about how they look. But prepare yourself for the fact that nothing you say will change their behavior—that is, nothing short of an extremely severe threat, which I do not recommend. An intense reaction on the part of the parent can increase a teenager's motivation to do something that is self-destructive simply to assert his own identity. On the other hand, adult acceptance of a teenager's differences might instill in the youngster a more casual and self-accepting attitude—and, in turn, inspire more constructive behavior.

I would much rather see parents focus their interest and criticism on issues of deeper concern and human values than on the way their children look. But while I don't feel that adults should openly interfere with a teenager's taste in clothing and hair style, I think you have a legitimate right to be concerned with cleanliness. In my experience, the best approach is to point out the possible consequences of poor hygiene: "If you continue to avoid a bath or shower, you are going to find it harder and harder to find friends who can tolerate the sight and smell of you." You are not then telling them what to do, but simply pointing out the possible results of their behavior.

Defiance and Bossiness

Our eight-year-old son used to be so well behaved—until several months ago when he became very bossy and quarrelsome, and now he refuses to listen to anything we tell him to do. I've been told that such a change is normal for a youngster of his age. Is this true?

It is not unusual for children to go through periodic and erratic changes in behavior. Generally, the negativistic and defiant stages occur when a child is around two years of age, again around the ages of seven and eight, and then again during the adolescent years. It sounds to me as if your son is attempting to show you how independent and self-assured he can be. It is up to you to try to channel his behavior into something more socially acceptable. You can do this by asking his advice about things and inviting him to express his feelings, rather than constantly *telling* him what to do. Focus on the things he does well, and you should find that his argumentative attitude will diminish.

Generally speaking, children at this age reflect some of their parents' own behavior, so you and your husband should examine your actions to see if he is in fact imitating or identifying with your way of dealing with things. If you yourselves are imperious instead of understanding, or inclined to bicker over small issues, you may find that an alteration in your behavior will lead to an alteration in his.

Bullying, Self-Defense, and Fighting Back

We've always told our five-year-old that fighting is wrong, and if another child hits him, he's not to hit back. But now, to our dismay, we discover that the other boys bully him—and he does little to resist. Please give us some guidelines! What do you tell a child about fighting under circumstances like this?

While children often imitate their parents' behavior, they also assimilate their values. You have obviously gotten across the idea that you consider fighting to be wrong. I agree with this attitude and feel that it's important to let children know that physical force and violence should not be used to intimidate other people. But when someone is actually being threatened or coerced and it is impossible to settle the situation with words, then physical self-defense is appropriate—and, I think, morally correct.

Encouraging your son to fight back when he is bullied by other youngsters is not inconsistent with your attitude about violence. Most children can easily understand the difference between being the aggressor, who provokes fights, and defending themselves when another person strikes first. Explain to your son that if he has done his best to avoid a skirmish, it may finally be necessary to defend himself. Let him know that even though you are proud of him for not hitting other children, you would understand if he absolutely *had* to hit to defend himself.

If you know that your child is being bullied by one or two other children on a regular basis, I see nothing wrong with intervening on your child's behalf. It may be necessary to contact the school if the bullying is taking place there, or to contact the other children's parents if it occurs elsewhere. By offering protection for your child, you will not make him a sissy but will affirm your role as a parent who is protective and loving.

The Child Who Bites

My two-year-old bites! When things aren't going his way or he gets into a scuffle with another child, he closes his teeth on the nearest fingers or arm. Is there a particular reason that a child does this? And how should I break him of the habit?

Two-year-olds are particularly primitive in the expression of their feelings. It is normal for them to grab, push, pull, and throw things, and periodically they become overwhelmed by frustration and indulge in temper tantrums. It is at this age that they attempt to assert their individuality and independence by acts of negativism and defiance. While all this is taking place, they are also trying to explore the environment and find what makes things happen. They are generally not capable of engaging in meaningful play with other small children for a sustained period of time. They are likely to engage instead in what we call "parallel play"—they play *alongside* other children rather than interact with others in a cooperative effort.

When children of this age become overwhelmed by their frustration, it is not too unusual for them to resort to biting. True, some children who are seriously emotionally disturbed often bite themselves as well as others. But most of the children who bite have not been taught firmly that this is totally unacceptable behavior. In your case, it is likely that your child's pattern of biting developed because you were not adamant enough the first few times he did it. I do not think you can "reason" with a two-year-old about such behavior. You must *show* your anger about this by your facial expression and your tone of voice. You may also have to resort to spanking, but I recommend this only if firmness does not suffice. Although some people disagree, I feel it is far better for a child to experience a mild spanking or a slap on the hand than it is for this kind of primitive behavior to continue. You should also immediately isolate your son from the situation in which he is playing or fighting, making it clear that he is not allowed to continue playing with others when he does this.

If your child seems unable to tolerate normal amounts of frustration, you may have to help him through this age period by diverting him from situations that are overwhelming and channeling his energies into activities where he can rid himself of anger without inflicting it on another person.

Handling Uncontrolled Aggression in Toddlers

I was sitting with other mothers in the playground recently when my son, who is two and a half, picked up his toy truck and hit another child with it. There was screaming and crying and apologizing (by me)—but my son didn't look repentant at all. Is this a sign of hostile or aggressive behavior that I should be concerned about?

Yes, this *is* a sign of hostility and aggression; although you should certainly be concerned about it, remember that such behavior is not at all uncommon in children between the ages of two and three. When going through this period—which is commonly called "the terrible twos"—children are clearly crude in the expression of their feelings. Most of them engage in what is called "parallel play," and they tend simply to grab things that they want from other children. Generally, they are three before they show the capacity for meaningful play with their peers.

While it is important for you to apologize for your son's act, I think it is more important for you to demonstrate—to him—your annoyance at his behavior. Let him know firmly that you are angry about what he did. This is neither the time nor the appropriate age to explain at great length and in an intellectual way the implications of his hostility—he will respond more appropriately to your emotional reaction than he will to your attempts to "reason" with him. Explain that if he continues to behave this way, you will not allow him to be with other children. Follow through on your threats. Your child will never develop a repentant attitude unless he understands that such behavior is unacceptable.

Arguing Openly in Front of the Family

My husband and I have a pact never to argue in front of the rest of the family—we think it's bad for the kids to see us angry with each other. Are we wrong to place such a premium on maintaining this facade of happiness and peace?

Children are taught to deal with life's problems by the experiences they have as they grow up, and the lessons they learn from those who love and protect them are usually the most impressive ones. In the course of life, children will be sure to see discord arise among those close to them. If they have never been exposed to such a situation, they may have feelings of guilt or self-deprecation when they themselves become angry or annoyed with someone they love.

If your children see that parents can argue heatedly and still love each other, they will gain much. You can teach them that the opposite of love is not hate but indifference. Moreover, parents are wasting their time if they think they are protecting their children—children are very sensitive to people's feelings and are usually only too aware of the façade.

I hasten to add that physical battles or name-calling sessions are not useful experience for children to witness (or for parents to participate in, for that matter). To the contrary, it is very frightening for a child to see that those he relies on for protection and security are out of control of themselves.

Protecting the Curious Toddler

Our three-year-old is so rambunctious and curious about everything that he's always banging himself up in his eagerness to do things. I constantly chase after him, cautioning him to be careful—but my husband says I should just leave him alone, that he's sturdy and won't hurt himself. Is he right?

If you've been successful in satisfying your son's emotional needs during infancy and early childhood, it is natural that his current quest for independence and individuality is now marked by increased mental or physical activity. Some children this age are outwardly more lively than others and tend to explore their ideas in a more physical way. Other children explore the world in a more mental way, through their fantasies; they pretend, they move around cautiously, they sometimes seem to be daydreaming. Your child is obviously one whose exploration of ideas happens to be more physical.

If you're convinced that your son's falls and minor injuries are not due to poor muscle coordination and if he seems free of emotional problems, you should, for the most part, take your husband's advice and give your child the freedom to move around spontaneously. It is, of course, necessary to protect him from obvious dangers, such as open windows, staircases, and similar hazards. But if you constantly nag him or warn him about every tiny potential danger, he will eventually begin to tune you out or may become so cautious that he will cling to you for fear that venturing away will have horrible consequences.

All children need some unobtrusive guidance and protection to develop their own sense of freedom and responsibility. In all likelihood, your eager and curious three-year-old needs an occasional reminder of potential hazards. However, a constant succession of reminders will convince him that, without your constant presence and protection, disaster is impending.

Children Who Run into the Street

Our four-year-old daughter ran directly into the path of a truck the other day as my husband and I were about to walk her across the very heavily trafficked street on which we live. How can we make her understand the danger involved in such an act without traumatizing her about crossing the street?

I'm sure you and your husband were appropriately traumatized by what your daughter did. Frankly speaking, if people lack anxiety about traffic and are not sufficiently fearful of the real dangers involved, they can get injured or even killed. I see nothing wrong with being "traumatized" about running into the street. This is one of those situations in life when I believe it's important to let a child know how intensely upset she has made you by running into the path of a truck. Let her know that she could have been killed or injured, and this could have not only been severely harmful to her but also would have left you extraordinarily upset. Let her know you love her very much and that's why you are so concerned about her welfare. When a child recognizes the intensity of a parent's feelings in situations like this, it offers reassurance to her or him about your feelings of love. Don't be the least hesitant about letting her know of your concern.

Stealing and Lying

My child is stealing. He comes home every day with something new, but he simply says other children have been giving him gifts. What should I do to make it clear that telling the truth is more important than anything else, and we will try to help him if he will only talk to us?

If your child claims that what he has in his possession is a gift from another child, he may be right, and your accusation of stealing can damage his trust in you. The first thing to do is to make sure that any accusations are based on fact. If, without embarrassing your child, you can contact the parents of the other child to determine the nature of the "exchange" of objects, it would serve you better in understanding the situation more fully and in working out the appropriate course of action.

If it turns out that he is stealing, it may help you to deal with the problem if you understand some of the common causes of stealing in children.

Chronic stealing and lying are frequently related to serious underlying emotional problems. Some young people never develop a sufficiently strong conscience or internalized values of what is right and what is wrong. They simply lie and steal without any feeling that it is wrong. It's extremely difficult to overcome this problem when a child gets much beyond five years of age if he or she has not developed these values in a strong and meaningful loving relationship with at least one parent who reflects certain ethical and moral social values. On the other hand, some children who know that stealing and lying are wrong continue to do so as a means of retaliation against authority: authorities like parents, toward whom—for reasons that require competent psychological assistance to uncover—they have very strong angry feelings.

Some children steal in the hope that they will get caught, which might embarrass their parents and, at the same time, lead the parents to give them the attention that they need. Some children, unfortunately, gain parental recognition only through socially unacceptable behavior and feel ignored when all is well. For other children, stealing is a way of acquiring objects that in some indirect way represent "supplies" of love and the kind of sustenance that is unconsciously related to the sense of strength or self-esteem. It's as if the objects they steal are a hedge against "emotional famine." These objects, in a way, counteract a feeling of loss within that person. If your child's stealing and lying are persistent or chronic, you should seek professional help.

All children at some time or other find objects they see as being extremely enticing and, as guilty as they may feel taking them, are overwhelmed by the desire to possess that object. Frequently the objects are displayed in an enticing way or are highly advertised or heavily promoted through the media. In instances like this, which may occur only occasionally, the "stealing" is more situational than basic to the child's personality. A child with a strong conscience may feel that what he or she has done is so wrong that it would be devastating to admit guilt; consequently that child may lie in the hope that the situation will dissipate itself and he or she will not have to face the embarrassment of admitting what has happened.

As far as punishment goes, I believe it's extremely important for parents to avoid being severely punitive when lying or stealing takes place, simply because it forces a child to feel you are mean and therefore makes the child feel self-righteous. That feeling of self-righteousness can then lead him to feel justified in stealing, and the lesson he's learned is that he'd better be careful next time to avoid getting caught. Milder forms of punishment have been shown in behavioral studies to be far more effective in helping the child develop a conscience about his behavior than severe forms of punishment. Under no circumstances should you treat your child as a criminal who has just committed grand larceny. Your behavior can be so devastating to the child that the ensuing loss of self-esteem can be so damaging and the hurt so great that your child will be fearful of you for a long time to come in a way that would interfere with any future communication.

Finally, no matter what punishment is decided on, it's important for all parents to make it clear to children that it is totally unacceptable to take things that belong to someone else. Tell them that they can get into trouble for doing this and it can cause them to lose friends. It's also important for parents to indicate that if a child steals, every effort should be made to tell the truth and return the object.

The "Me First" Syndrome

Whenever my six-year-old son and four-year-old daughter play a game together, the older child insists on winning—or on playing the games and rules he sets. He must be the first in everything—going up stairs, having his choice of hamburgers or toys, ordering the first ice-cream cone. Our younger child doesn't seem to mind as yet, but we don't like this overly dominant attitude in our son. What can we do to curtail it without making him even more stubborn?

It sounds as if your six-year-old doesn't feel secure unless he is "first," or, in a sense, the "*only one*." Being the winner, in his mind, may be the equivalent of being the only one. Remember, he *was* the only one until he was two years of age, when his sister was born. At that point he may have had doubts about his position in the family, which caused him to need constant reassurance that he is accepted. His greatest feeling of emotional security may have been when he was the only child. He has attempted to recapture that feeling by fighting to be "first."

In my experience, this kind of struggle to be in first place occurs much more often, and with greater intensity, when children are around two or two and a half years apart in age. Children who are around two years of age are somewhat crude in the expression of their feelings and require substantially more parental time and attention than they do when they are perhaps three years of age or older.

It seems evident to me that your six-year-old's competitive spirit has been "fueled" by the two-year age difference between himself and his sister.

Your son is not being as dominant as he is being anxious. His anxiety seems based on his fear of losing parental love and affection. If you give him more love and affection, as well as some undivided attention, you may find that his competitiveness will subside spontaneously. It would help matters if you explained to him, during those times when communication between you and him is best, that you love him very much and that your love is undiminished, even when he doesn't win games or is second, third, or even the loser. Try to get across the idea that being first, or winning, has nothing whatsoever to do with your love and acceptance of him.

It would also be helpful if, when he loses a game or is prevented from being first in ordering his ice cream or hamburger, that you help him cope with his anxiety by showing him, at that moment, that you love him. It doesn't have to be with words—in fact it's better communicating with a hug, a reassuring look, or even a kiss. Finally, without being harsh, you can set certain ground rules about going upstairs or placing food orders that serves to minimize the number of situations where his drive to be first will occur.

"I Hate You"

I'm beginning to wonder if my daughter really loves me. Every once in a while she screams, "I hate you!" Whenever she says it, she's always very angry and I know she means what she says by the expression on her face and the tone of her voice. Most of the time she acts as all other children do and seems to enjoy my company, wants me to read to her at bedtime, and is eager to tell me about her accomplishments at school. Nevertheless, it still disturbs me to hear her scream, "I hate you!" Is it possible that she actually means it?

No one ever loves another person all the time no matter how deep a loving bond there is. There are bound to be periods of frustration, and this frustration leads to anger. In fact, when the feeling of love is very deep for another person, any frustration in that loving relationship can perhaps raise more intense anger than it would in a relationship with little deep feeling. Anger and love are feelings that are in a way related to each other. Not caring at all, or feeling indifferent, is distinctly different from these other intense emotions. Understandably, your daughter gets angry and expresses her feelings very directly when she feels you do not comply with her expectations or satisfy her feelings. She is able to vent her feelings with you without feeling any threat of the loss of your love for doing so. I believe it's important for people to be able to express their pent-up emotions to avoid developing the kind of internalized pressure that causes them to explode in destructive ways. At the same time, I don't believe we should encourage or allow people to express their feelings in a way that destroys the integrity of other people or is harmful to them with the justification that it's important to get rid of unpleasant feelings. Children frequently find it easier to express their feelings directly to a parent, since they are basically assured of parental love and know that they will not be rejected for their directness.

As a general rule, parents should encourage their children to express their feelings *verbally* so that these feelings can be further discussed and resolved constructively. I don't approve of children being allowed to destroy objects or lash out physically and hit their parents. It's absolutely essential for a child to learn to come to terms with angry feelings in a way that allows for the release of these feelings, but in a socially acceptable way. And the best place for this to take place is in the home and in the security of a loving relationship between you and your children. From all that you say about your daughter, it sounds to me as if she has a deep love for you and feels secure enough in her relationship with you that she can vent her feelings and still be assured of your love for her.

Gangs and Bullies

I found out my daughter is a member of a gang whose sole purpose is to pick on another smaller group of kids. How can I keep her from joining in these awful activities?

I believe you have a right to be annoyed with her for engaging in an activity such as this. Make it clear to her that you have no objections to her having friends who are united in activities that are helpful or useful to other people or whose purpose it is to participate in some activity that does not infringe upon the rights of others, but that you totally disapprove of this kind of bullying and harassment. Let her know that people who feel weak and frightened within themselves sometimes gang together to show their strength to people weaker or smaller than they. Let her know at the same time that you love her and respect many of the things she does but that you are totally against this kind of activity.

I think that you should also take it upon yourself to contact the parents of some of her gang members and discuss their feelings about what the children are doing. You might suggest, not only to your daughter but to the parents of her friends, that perhaps she and her friends can do something that's worthwhile for people who need help rather than cause harm to other people and put them in a position where they're intimidated. I believe parents should guide children—not push them—toward ways in which they can help people and gain recognition through good deeds.

Somewhere along the line you should ask your daughter to pretend that she is one of the younger children being intimidated. Ask her to tell you how she would feel if she were in his or her place. Don't hesitate to emphasize that what they are doing is cruel, something to be ashamed of, and something which in no way reflects strength of character.

My child will only play with one friend, no matter how many children I introduce him to. There are twenty other children in his class. How can I get him to show an interest in other children?

You simply offer him the opportunity to get to know these other children better by expressing the willingness to have them come and visit your home. Apparently you've done this and your child still prefers to play with one friend. I see absolutely nothing wrong with this. He apparently enjoys focusing his interest on one friend rather than spreading himself out among many. In all likelihood he and his friend are sufficiently compatible to meet each other's needs at this particular time.

Children frequently sense this kind of compatibility and understandably can prefer a deeper relationship with one person. In many ways your child is showing a capacity for deeper friendship than if he were to bounce from child to child or look upon his contacts with classmates in a more scattered way. In all likelihood, he will develop other friendships in time, perhaps in the same way he's developed this friendship—that is, by devoting his time and interest to one person at a time. If you examine your own childhood, you will probably find that you had a "best friend" and you felt that that friendship would last forever. Inevitably, another person came along and took that first friend's place.

Children are also temperamentally different. Some will always prefer a one-to-one relationship while others prefer relating to a wider range of friends. From a psychological viewpoint, there is nothing wrong with either approach. I believe that parents should recognize the individuality of a child and provide him or her with every opportunity to foster good friendship in whatever style the child prefers. It's most important that you respect your child's integrity and dignity and not coerce him into weakening his ties with his one friend in order to fulfill your wish for him to have a greater range of friends.

The Demanding Child During Illness

My child has been quite ill recently. We have had to stay close to his bedside, and whenever he wanted anything to eat or drink we rushed to get it because it was so important that he get some nourishment. Now that he is well again, he is every bit as demanding and difficult as during his illness. How can we bring him back to the everyday world?

When children are seriously ill, they understandably become anxious and so do their parents. This anxiety leads to greater vigilance on everyone's part and causes parents and health professionals to give more and better care to that child than he would receive if he were healthy. This is not only a sensible response but quite appropriate to the child's physical and mental health. Needless to say, the emotional comfort a child gets from this kind of attention is very easy to live with. His desire to keep it going is not unlike what your response would be if you checked into a very luxurious hotel and took advantage of all the coddling and room service you'd have at your fingertips. The fact of the matter is you have to learn to get back to the real world eventually and so does he.

Let him know you understand that he was anxious and upset during his illness and that he needed greater care than he usually gets to make him healthy and well again. Explain that he had gotten used to it and that you don't blame him for wanting to keep it going—after all, anyone would with the kind of care he had gotten! Once you've explained this to him, it should be easier for him to accept this kind of response on your part when he becomes demanding: "You can do that yourself now —you're no longer sick." Don't expect him to make his adjustment overnight, but if you continue to point this out and encourage him to use his own resources, both he and you will enjoy not only his return to health but his return to greater self-sufficiency.

Defiance and Punishment

I warned my child three times that she should come home directly from school and yet I found out that she stopped over at a friend's house for an hour and did not even apologize when she finally meandered in the front door. What kind of punishment would be appropriate for a child who repeatedly ignores warnings?

To begin with, perhaps you are being too demanding about restricting her visits to a friend after school. You might suggest that you like her to come home directly from school but that if she stops at a friend's, it's absolutely essential that she telephone you so that you know where she is. In this way, you're giving her more freedom of movement but at the same time showing your concern for her and setting a rule that enables her to function more independently without causing you undue anguish. When parents are too demanding with children and set severe limits on their freedom of movement, children can become extremely compliant, never show any expression of their own, and become fearful about challenging authority. On the other hand, the child may defy you completely and disregard any rules and regulations you set up. In order for you to have your child respect your wishes, ideas, rules, and regulations, it's important for you to show respect for your child's individuality and to recognize what her wishes and desires are even if you can't comply with them. When there's open communication between parents and children based upon mutual respect of each other's wishes and feelings, it's far easier to resolve these problems than if communication is severely restricted.

Nevertheless, if a punishment becomes appropriate when a child continually defies a parent's rules and regulations, the punishment should be appropriate to the "crime," both in time proximity and in severity. To deprive a child of the treat of going to the circus with his classmates three months hence because he failed to make his bed one day is not only extremely severe but too far away in the future and not at all consistent with his wrongdoing. I believe that parents should consult their children about the appropriateness of punishment when they violate the rules. For example, explain to your child, "I warned you that I would have to punish you if you did it again—you did, and now we have to decide upon a punishment. What do *you* think a reasonable punishment would be for what you've done that's wrong?" More often than not, children recommend a punishment that is extremely severe and one that no parent would care to enforce. I recall one child saying to me when presented with the option to decide on punishment, "Don't feed me for a month!" You continue to negotiate by saying, "That's too severe. Think of another one." You can ultimately find something that shows you are not only strong in enforcing the rule but that you are compassionate in not wanting it to be too severe. Moreover, by taking into consideration the child's wishes and feelings, you are showing respect for him. A child will tend to accept a reasonable punishment in a more noble manner than if the punishment is severe and administered in a dispassionate way.

Bickering Among Children

Would you please tell me how to handle kids who are constantly quarreling and fighting? My children are six, eight, and eleven, and things are at a stage of total warfare in our family.

Intense and frequent quarreling among siblings is often a sign that the children feel short-changed, that each feels the others are depriving him or her of parental attention. And the harassed parent who tries to convince the children that they are "all loved exactly the same" may find that this impersonal reassurance makes things even worse.

It is best if you treat siblings as individuals right from the start, making clear that each one is a different person with different needs. I recommend that parents give each of their children some concentrated attention—perhaps once or twice a week—as if he or she were the only one that counted at that time. It's not the *amount* of time that is of primary concern; it's the fact that the time belongs to this patricular child and is geared to his specific interests and ccncerns.

One last point: There is a specific factor that often contributes to the sort of situation you describe. If parents compare one child to another—"Look how nicely Ricky cleans his room. Why can't you do the same?"—it invariably causes hostility toward the child who makes the others look "unacceptable." This resentment can result in inordinate amounts of friction among children.

Acting Up in Special Situations

I took my six-year-old—who usually is bright and polite—to an interview at the school I hope she'll be attending next year. In front of the principal, she reverted to infantile behavior and was barely able to answer his simplest question. I was horribly embarrassed. And we were no sooner out the door than she was talking away intelligently and happily again. Why on earth did she act this way? I had told her the night before that this was an important occasion and that she should be on her best behavior.

I am sure that every parent has lived through an experience similar to yours. Sometimes when you want your children to be functioning at their best, they act their worst. But children are sensitive and often respond to aspects of a situation that you may not even be aware of. The fact that she was being evaluated, your embarrassment and concern over this matter—anything could have caused her to become tense, constricted, and defensive.

Since you know your six-year-old to be communicative, intelligent, and generally happy, my conclusion is that she was simply responding to a stressful situation. The fact that you warned your daughter the night before that this was an "important occasion" requiring her "best behavior" may have added to the emotional tension. As a general rule, I think it's best for parents to prepare their children for an interview such as this by explaining what will occur and by offering them emotional support. If your daughter had been given sufficient time to establish a relationship with a trusted adult—in this case the interviewing principal—it is more than likely that her true nature would have been revealed.

Head Banging

I have a fourteen-month-old son, and when he gets upset, he starts hitting his head on the closet wall or solid object. Is it normal for him to do this? And how should I deal with it when it happens?

Generally speaking, it is not normal for young children—or any children, for that matter—to hit their heads on hard objects when they become frustrated. Sometimes children hurt themselves by accident when having a temper tantrum, but if time after time they continue to engage in self-destructive behavior, it is generally a sign that they are overwhelmed by aggressive tendencies that they are unable to deal with.

When children are frustrated, it is necessary for them to drain off the resultant hostility in some way. Generally their aggression is channeled outward to some object or person in their environment, but if such outlets are blocked, the child may have no choice but to direct his rage in toward himself.

It has been my experience over the years that some children who feel unimportant to their parents—and, therefore, insignificant in general—may engage in self-destructive behavior such as you describe. I suggest that you do your best to minimize the amount of frustration your child encounters and attempt to reassure and comfort him when he does become frustrated. If the symptom is not relieved by these efforts, then I feel that it *may* reflect an underlying emotional problem, and I urge you to seek professional help. While it may be difficult to diagnose a disorder when a child is this young, at least some initial consultation and periodic follow-up will help you to know as time passes whether or not this is a serious problem.

Childhood Destructiveness

Do all children like to destroy things deliberately? My four-year-old daughter and her friend just crawled under the seats of her father's new boat and picked away chunks of the Styrofoam flotation material. She also ruins her toys by taking them apart, and yesterday I found her peeling off patches of wallpaper! Are these destructive tendencies normal?

There are some things, which I call "invitational lures," that absolutely destroy a child's self-control. I am sure you have had various temptations like hers. When you see peeling wallpaper, don't *you* have an urge to pull it off even more? For a four-year-old such temptations are far greater. And mixed with an intense curiosity about what makes things work, some of these "destructive tendencies" are impossible to resist. A child is also influenced greatly by the behavior of other children. If she finds another little boy or girl doing something destructive, it is very tempting to join in the same activity.

While it is important to understand these situations from a child's point of view, it is equally important for you to set limits on what is acceptable behavior and what is not. You will have to affirm and reaffirm those limits periodically—and prepare yourself for the fact that your child will at times ignore them. Be consistent, and let your child know that if she continues to do these things you prohibit, you will have to punish her. If your punishment is appropriate and not overly severe, she will begin to incorporate your values into her life and, in this way, begin to develop internalized controls over her own behavior.

Sharing and Respecting Personal Property

My children are always fighting over each other's possessions, and invariably my younger son borrows his brother's toys and breaks them or loses pieces to a game. My older son becomes furious and retaliates. How can I stop the warfare between them over their possessions and teach them how to share and yet how to respect each other's property?

In some families this is an extremely difficult problem to resolve simply because the children are very close in age and each child is greatly enticed by the possessions of the other. When children are further apart in age, their interests usually vary sufficiently for them to have little interest in one another's games or belongings.

While it's impossible for me to explain how you should deal specifically with your children, let me suggest some guidelines that you can adapt to your own family situation by using words you're comfortable with and which are understandable to your children. To begin with, don't try to establish ground rules for solving this problem while tempers are high. When all is well between your children and no conflict is at hand, let them know that you would like each of them to be able to borrow belongings from one another, enjoy them, and return them in good condition. Let them know you want them to respect each other as well as each other's properties and that life would be best for everyone if this can be done without arguments, destructiveness, and retaliation. Ask them how *they* think the rules should be set up to accomplish your goal. Try to keep your discussion on the issue of borrowing and try to avoid any personal accusations by one against the other. Remarks such as, "He always breaks my things; I never ever break any of his things," should be dealt with by your pointing out that you now want to work arrangements out to protect the rights of each. The more you get your children involved in setting up the rules, the easier it will be for them to follow through on these rules, and it certainly puts you in a position where you can remind them that these are their rules and not your rules.

Once you've established rules that seem to be agreeable to everyone, you then have to work out a plan to deal with violations of these rules. Punishment and reparations are necessary if you are to be in a position where these rules are enforced. Again, ask for their suggestions but be prepared with a backup set of your own, since young people are frequently more harsh in recommended punishment than adults might be. Perhaps you might suggest that if one breaks or loses something that belongs to the other that it be replaced by funds drawn from a weekly allowance. Frankly speaking, this can be too heavy a financial burden for any child, and you might want to work out a formula where you pay half the damages when they occur. While this might seem like an injustice for you, I believe it's a part of parenthood and one of those responsibilities that come with teaching your child how to handle problems.

While this solution will not work all of the time, in my experience it communicates the important issues involved in borrowing, losing, and returning belongings of others, and encourages greater respect for other people's property or discourages them from borrowing things promiscuously.

Trading Possessions

For our eight-year-old son's birthday, we gave him a nice lunchbox that he seemed to like very much. But the other day he came home from school without it—he said he'd "traded it" to another boy in exchange for some comic books. I don't know exactly what to do about this—it was his lunchbox. Do children have a right to give away their possessions as they please? Or should I make him get the lunchbox back?

Theoretically, children should have the right to give away their possessions if they please. But every effort should be made through parental guidance to help the child see as objectively as possible the implications of his or her generosity as well as the consequences.

In your case, concerning a lunchbox, the problem is a little bit more complicated. Obviously, your child is showing independence and assertiveness. This creates a paradox for you, since I'm sure you want to encourage this kind of behavior but at the same time protect him from giving up a possession which is more like a household item than a toy. What complicates the problem is the fact that it was a birthday gift and not a possession bought in the vein of a household item.

Let me suggest that you point out the fact that in *your* judgment he should not have traded something like this for comic books but perhaps something else in the same category. However, because he has now done it he will now have to carry his lunch to school in a paper bag. This may provide sufficient inconvenience for him to recognize the folly of his decision. If he finds this to be inconvenient and is remorseful about having traded his lunchbox for comic books, you might consider getting him another lunchbox but not immediately. Give him a week or two of carrying his lunch to school in a paper bag so that the inconvenience becomes an important enough experience that he will give more consideration in the future concerning the implications of his trades. In this way, you will be recognizing and accepting his independence, offering him guidance for the future, allowing him sufficient inconvenience to make him more thoughtful, and at the same time showing him that you are considerate enough of "errors" like this so that you are willing to offer him some help in making his life more convenient again—it makes you an understanding parent.

Whining

My six-year-old daughter nags and whines constantly about every little thing—she wants mustard on her sandwich, she doesn't want mustard on her sandwich—on and on and on until I am at my wit's end and I feel like screaming. Why do children whine like this? And how should a parent deal with it? Our three-year-old daughter doesn't seem to be a whiner at all.

In a sense, children who whine endlessly about little things have been encouraged to do so—often by the very adults who find his behavior so upsetting. It is natural that parents sometimes lose patience and give in to a pleading child simply to make things easier for themselves at the moment. If your child's whining does stop when you give her what she wants, it seems likely that you unknowingly have reinforced this very pattern that bothers you.

The fact that your three-year-old doesn't act in this manner suggests that she is able to accomplish her goals in other ways. But when your younger child was first born, in all likelihood your older daughter saw you respond to her newborn sister when she cried and fussed. Consciously or unconsciously, she may have learned that you were quick to react when crying occurred, and she too may have adopted this characteristic way of gaining your attention. The fact that she is so fussy and demanding about little things also suggests that she still may feel as if her little sister gets more of your time and attention than she does.

I suggest you absolutely avoid giving her what she wants when she whines. Make it clear that you will not fulfill any of her demands if she uses such a tone of voice. Listen to her carefully when she tries to communicate with you calmly, and carry out some of her wishes when she speaks to you without whining—and she should quickly learn that she can accomplish her purposes more readily if she does not nag and fuss.

Dealing with Crying Infants

We know that you strongly advocate picking up crying babies at all hours of the day and night, and we do our best to follow your advice. But our nine-month-old son wakes up in the middle of the night and cries and cries until we come to play. Is this normal? How should we deal with him?

As babies approach ten or eleven months of age they may indeed wake up at night and attempt to have fun. Obviously, this should not be encouraged. Let your baby know that you are there, but make it clear that you have no intention of socializing in the middle of the night. Do this by putting the child down firmly in his bed and comforting him by patting his back. If he pulls himself up, put him down again —without getting angry—and make it clear that this is bedtime. You may find that your child will pull himself up many times before getting the message that you are not going to play at that hour, and each time he does pull himself up, put him back gently but quite firmly on his stomach to go to sleep.

My four-year-old son is a sensitive child, and I encourage him to cry and express his feelings. However, my husband insists that we should not support our son when he weeps over what my husband calls "every little thing." Is my husband right about this?

Children should indeed be allowed to express their feelings, and they are inclined to do so with people whom they trust. However, merely expressing one's feelings is not enough. It's important to learn how to cope with the problems that *cause* unpleasant feelings in order to gain a sense of mastery over some of life's stresses. I have seen parents who encourage their children to express their feelings as a catharsis but then never follow up with guidance—and these children turn out to be very anxious and sometimes even more upset because they have been left "hanging." They have learned no lessons about utilizing their own resources to resolve the problem situation itself.

Tears are certainly appropriate in many situations, and they should not be limited solely to a female. If each time your child cries, however, he gains some recognition from you that is not forthcoming in any other way, weeping will become one way of showing that he needs you. It is possible that he is weeping over "every little thing"—but the message behind his tears may be, "Please pay attention to me even when I don't cry."

I have a twenty-two-month-old daughter. When she's hurt or upset or just wants attention, my husband will immediately tell her to stop crying. It's hard for me to see her fighting to hold back her sobs. Is she being hurt by this treatment?

At twenty-two months of age, it is hard for children to articulate their needs. If you can provide comfort and gratification at this time, you will ease your child forward into the period when she *can* express herself in words—and crying will become a less important means of conveying discomfort. In fact, children who continue such prolonged crying in later years are those who found little gratification of their needs during this preverbal stage.

If your daughter is forced to hold back her tears, this will prevent her from expressing her true feelings and will encourage her to bottle up her emotions—and this could be the start of an emotional pattern that could set off great inner tension in years to come. There is another factor: children, and grownups as well, often develop physical symptoms when they are unable to express their feelings in a spontaneous manner. I have seen many patients who were discouraged from crying by their parents who later developed a pattern of chronic colds and other respiratory disturbances, such as allergic and hay-fever reactions (a person who has a cold is very much like someone who has just gotten over a crying episode).

In short, if crying is suppressed, a person may manifest the symptoms of crying in other ways, both physical and mental.

If our baby wails and I'm pretty sure there's nothing wrong with him, I'm inclined to let him cry it out. But my husband invariably ends up cuddling the baby until he's quiet. Doesn't this mean we're likely to have a spoiled child on our hands?

Absolutely not—no baby is spoiled by cuddling. The fact that your husband's attentions ultimately quiet the baby means that the infant needed this attention to change its emotional state from one of fear, rage, and discomfort to one of comfort, pleasure, and trust.

Studies have shown that babies like to experience a variety of sensory stimulation. An infant's developing nervous system seems to thrive on the nourishment of different sights and sounds and touches—and your cuddling and attention provide this stimulation. It also gives your baby a sense of trust in the environment and in people. The baby whose cries are answered now will later be the child confident enough to show his independence and curiosity. But the baby who is left to cry it out may develop a sense of isolation and distrust and may turn inward by turning out the world that will not answer its cry. And later on in life, this child may continue to cope with stress by trying to shut out reality.

Reasoning, Discipline, and the Young Child

We have friends who reason with their five-year-old son and explain in great detail—"why it makes Mommy unhappy when he pours milk on the floor" and so forth. Is this a wise procedure to use when disciplining a child? Should a youngster of this age be given extensive reasons for rules his parents make?

I would agree that explaining in detail to a two-year-old would probably prove fruitless. When children are as old as five, however, it is important for parents to explain as best they can *why* they are unhappy or angry. When milk is poured on the floor, Mommy or Daddy must clean it up, and a child should be able to understand why this annoys his parents.

But whatever the age of the child, perhaps the most important thing is that parents demonstrate their feelings rather than merely recite statements about their displeasure. It is fairly meaningless to explain in a controlled, dispassionate way your reasons for being upset. Clearly *showing* that annoyance by the tone of your voice and the firmness of your actions is far more effective. And the expression of your feelings, accompanied by a literal explanation, helps children to feel, as well as intellectually understand, the consequences of their actions.

Following Through on Threats

I have a six-year-old daughter who laughs at me when I discipline her or lecture her. Should I be more forceful? She seems not to care at all.

Being forceful may not solve your problem. She obviously defies the rules and regulations you set up and in all likelihood this occurs because you do not follow through on the promises and threats you make. I see this frequently in parents who say things like "If I find you leaving your games all over the floor, I'm going to throw them out!" and who never follow through on their threats. I don't believe that parents should make threats if they are not going to carry them out, any more than I believe they should make promises that they fail to carry out. This causes children to doubt what their parents say, and in many ways it shatters the parent's credibility to the child. In my experience I find that when parents are inconsistent in this way, children tend to be more defiant of rules and regulations, almost as if they are saying to the parent, "Please show me that you are consistent—I don't believe you are going to carry out your threats or promises." In a way, they are asking you to stop them and hope you will show the strength of your convictions. When a parent means what he or she says, it provides a child with a greater feeling of security than when a parent makes idle or extreme assertions and threats that never are fulfilled. Your six-year-old probably doesn't believe you mean what you say, or doesn't feel that you care enough about her behavior to carry out and enforce the rules and regulations you have set up.

Discipline and Eating Habits

My grandchildren are allowed to leave the dinner table even though there is food on their plates. It makes me cringe—my children had to eat everything or they could not leave, no matter how they fussed. I remind my daughter of this and she just laughs and says it's not important. Am I terribly old-fashioned?

This really depends on a family's lifestyle. Some people feel that children should be forced to eat everything on their plates, but this can make mealtime unpleasant and take all the joy out of eating with others, so I am inclined to agree with your daughter. However, I do feel that some ground rules for eating should be established when young children are verbal enough to understand and discuss these matters. For example, I think it is fair to insist that a child taste new foods but not necessarily eat full portions of them. And while I think it right to urge a child to finish the food that he or she has asked for, I don't think any psychologically useful point is made by insisting that the child finish *everything* on his or her plate.

Eating Problems

For several weeks now, my fifteen-month-old child has been spitting out just about any kind of food I try to give her, and I'm becoming very alarmed about the whole thing. Is it awful for me to force-feed her?

Yes, it would be horrible for you to force-feed your child. You would only make the feeding experience an unpleasant one and reinforce your child's adverse reaction to it.

The fact is that many children go through stages where they eat very little but seem to grow perfectly normally. As long as your pediatrician is satisfied with your child's health and growth, I don't think you have anything to worry about.

It is possible that your fifteen-month-old has been spitting out food because of her growing sense of independence and the need to assert herself. Try giving her "finger foods"—things like bits of fruit, flakes of cereal, small pieces of meat, and other tidbits that she can pick up and put in her mouth herself. Also, give her more of the things that she seems to like and less of the things she spits out. And then, as a relaxed atmosphere is reestablished at mealtime, your child should become more and more willing to experiment with other foods that will give her a more balanced diet.

Junk Food

My two sons eat corn chips, potato chips, and cookies by the dozen, but their lunchboxes come home from school each day untouched. I beg them to tell me what they would like to eat for lunch, but they won't answer. I am worried that their terrible eating habits are damaging their physical health? What should I do?

There is absolutely no way you can keep your child from eating junk foods from time to time. It's easy for nutritionists to advise people to keep them away from children, but when you're a parent whose children associate with other children and where these foods are abundantly available, it's extremely difficult, if not impossible, to avoid the problem. My own personal view, and I'm *not* a nutritionist, is that you should do whatever you can to limit your child's intake of poor foods without becoming a harsh and depriving parent. To begin with, don't buy them. Secondly, buy foods in the same category that *are* nutritious and lack the food additives you want them to avoid. Experience tells me that children enjoy fresh fruit and raw vegetables such as carrots, celery, green peppers, and cucumbers. If these become part of your diet and are inserted in their lunchboxes, perhaps you'll be able to curb a good deal of their consumption of those foods you're trying to avoid. Bear in mind that it's impossible to avoid the problem altogether but continue to convey your attitudes and values while substituting as much as possible these foods for nutritionally sound ones. Many parents I know who object to children eating these "unacceptable" foods have them at home where they're easily acquired by their children. It always seems ironic to me that parents would buy things that they don't want their children to consume. I also think it's important for you to make sure that the other two meals your children eat at home—breakfast and dinner—are sufficiently balanced nutritionally to compensate for those meals your child eats at school.

The Overweight Child

My daughter, who is ten, has been overweight for several years now. I constantly remind her of her diet and her father teases her about being "tubby"—and we end up having terrible arguments. Are there reasons why she eats as much as she does? Is our relationship being damaged by our insistence that she stick to her diet?

Some children are overweight because of a medical problem, such as a metabolic disorder. Have your child checked carefully by your doctor to make sure there is no health problem contributing to her condition. If there is no physical basis for her inordinate appetite, then you might consider a psychological evaluation to see if her eating is due to an emotional problem. People who eat insatiably often make an unconscious association between the intake of food and the feeling of being loved, since in early infancy love and attention were part of the feeding process.

Some children are sufficiently concerned about

their obesity to want help and will often welcome paternal guidelines for a realistic diet. If the help is offered in a constructive manner, children are much more likely to accept it than if it is done in a punitive or depriving manner. Ridiculing children can only serve to increase their feelings of inadequacy —which might in turn cause them to eat more in defiance of their parents or as a means of gaining emotional gratification. You already know that your arguments with your daughter are futile. Continuing these arguments and insisting that she stick to her diet when she seems unable to do so can indeed damage your relationship. If this pattern continues, I would certainly recommend that you seek psychological help to come to terms with this problem.

Parental Outbursts of Rage

I have a very hot temper, and when my sons (they're ages eleven, nine, and eight) start to bicker and fight, I usually blow up and yell and scream. When I calm down, I always tell them I love them and didn't mean to upset them, and they always forgive me, but I worry that these outbreaks of mine will hurt them emotionally. Am I damaging them?

I am sure your persistent outbreaks are not doing any real good. However, they should not lead to any irreparable emotional damage as long as it is clear that your outrage is caused by your inflammable temperament and not by their unforgivable behavior. Since you do acknowledge their feelings and apologize, it is not likely that your sons are harboring excessive feelings of guilt that could hurt them later on. Their forgiving attitude certainly indicates that you all seem to have a good relationship. In fact, situations like this may even help children to understand and cope with other people's moods. (I am not, however, recommending that parents lose their tempers simply to teach their children this kind of lesson!)

Try discussing this matter with your sons. Explain to them how much you hate losing your temper and how much more pleasant it would be if they could avoid the bickering and fighting that cause you to flare up. A frank and open discussion should result in a more concerted effort on their part to prevent the circumstances that set off such scenes in the first place.

Parental Avoidance of Discipline

My husband does not believe in disciplining our four children—they've always done as they wished. Now our oldest son has dropped out of high school and is in trouble with the law. Is this because he's always been treated with such leniency?

It is very difficult to attribute your son's problems solely to this one factor. I will say, however, that it is important for every child to have a concerned father who actively participates in the family unit. And this participation needs to include evidence of the father's tenderness and love, as well as a firmness and control that shows he is really concerned about his youngster's welfare. The father who uses discipline to enforce consistent and reasonable rules of behavior conveys the feeling that he really cares about his children.

The parent who avoids disciplining his children

in order to be known as a "good father" is more concerned with his popularity than he is with his child's needs and healthy emotional development. The child whose father is weak, ineffectual, or inconsistent may be deprived of a strong figure to identify with, and may have difficulty dealing with authority as he grows older.

Discussing a Child's Problems When He's Around

Is it right to talk about young children's problems when they're around? My six-year-old daughter has been having some persistent problems in school, and I often discuss this with other parents even though she's playing in the room. She never seems to be paying attention —she'll be off in a corner with her dollhouse or something—and it's only lately that a friend has suggested that she hears and is bothered by what I say. Do children pick up this sort of thing?

Absolutely! Children are influenced by everything that happens to them, and hearing you talk about her problems is certainly going to affect her. People should apply the same standards to children that they apply to anyone else in matters like this. Imagine how you would feel if you overheard someone speculating on your life as though you were not even there.

Hearing you discuss her problems in this way can cause your daughter to feel unimportant, different, and even stigmatized—and indicates that you think she is incapable of understanding what you are talking about. Many children have told me that their parents "don't understand them," and your unintentional lack of consideration for her feelings is precisely the kind of thing that could cause a child to feel this. If this is the case, her problems in school may be at least partly due to your lack of insight into her needs, wishes, and feelings. Perhaps you ought to speak with a professional about your relationship in an effort to get to the bottom of her difficulties.

Discipline—When Parents Disagree

The other day I told my nine-year-old he couldn't watch television until he had completed his homework—and minutes later I discovered him in front of the set because "Dad said" he could watch it. This happens all the time. I'll do my best to discipline the children, and my husband will blithely counteract my orders. Is this sort of thing good for the kids?

Absolutely not. While it isn't necessary for parents to agree on all aspects of a child's discipline and punishment, it is extremely important that one not undermine the authority of the other. When parents contradict each other on a disciplinary matter such as this, the child is left feeling vulnerable and insecure because of the inconsistencies he encounters. Also, the child's loyalty is torn: which parent should he obey?

Even if the father feels that the mother is unjust in her demands, it is best if he temporarily supports her position. Later, both can talk it over in private and strike a compromise about the "united front" both should take. If by chance one parent still insists on the "rightness" of his or her stand, he might comment on the compromised position by telling the children, "You may feel this is unfair, but it is important to do what Mother asks. You may not like it, but that's the way life is at times."

On some occasions we find it necessary to discipline our five-year-old by spanking her—and after the punishment is over, she looks so downcast that I take her in my arms and tell her everything is all right. My husband says that this weakens the punishment and we shouldn't comfort her. Is he right?

To begin with, I would like to distinguish between discipline and punishment. Discipline, in my mind, means the establishment of rules and regulations of behavior set up to protect oneself and the rights of others. Punishment is the price you pay for violating these rules.

As far as punishment is concerned, I firmly believe it is best to warn children in advance of a spanking. "If you do this one more time, I am afraid I will have to spank you." If your child does misbehave again, you should carry out your promise, but the spanking should not be harsh. Taking your child into your arms after a spanking does not weaken the punishment—*provided* you explain, "I do not like to spank you and it upset me to do so, but you disobeyed me and it was necessary." However, if you simply hold her and tell her everything is all right, you are contradicting yourself, because it was *not* all right. By making it clear that you spanked her because you were annoyed with her but at the same time you still love her, she will learn a very important lesson in life—that it is possible to love someone and still be angry with them periodically without undermining that feeling of love.

We have a bright, thirteen-month-old little girl. Often when she is reprimanded, she becomes so frustrated that she attempts to hit us. We feel that by tapping her bottom or hands we would be participating in the very behavior we object to—and yet we feel these angry flails demand some sort of response from us. How should we handle the situation? Should we spank her?

It is not at all unusual for a child of your daughter's age to show her overwhelming frustration in this way, and if you understand that this is normal, it should be easier for you to deal with. However, I think you should make it clear that while you do not object to her *feelings* of anger and annoyance, you will not allow her to hit you.

I agree that by hitting her back you would be engaging in precisely the behavior you're trying to discourage. Instead of spanking her, even in the mildest way, take her by the arms, hold her, and explain in a very firm and annoyed tone of voice that you do *not* want her to hit you. While she may not literally understand your words, the firmness of your voice and your grip will let her know of your determination. After you have gotten your message across (and this should take only seconds), you can release her so that she knows she is not being permanently restrained.

While I am not totally opposed to an occasional spanking, I do not feel that this situation calls for it. I feel that spanking should be limited to those times when a child is literally doing something that endangers life or health and an immediate and strong parental response is necessary. A spanking may also be appropriate in other circumstances—for instance, when a child ignores all parental efforts at enforcing rules—provided the parent warns in advance that if the unacceptable behavior continues, a spanking will be forthcoming. In any event, I do not feel that the spanking should ever be more than a mild one, since its main purpose is to convey the parents' disapproval of certain behavior and their consistency in enforcing the limits that they have set.

Discipline and the Stepparent

My husband's fourteen-year-old daughter from his previous marriage left last week after visiting us for a month. As patient as I tried to be, I found her incredibly demanding and headstrong. Her father lets her do anything she wants, and when I try to reprimand her, everybody looks at me as if I were an old witch. Are there any guidelines you can give me for the next visit?

You must take into consideration the fact that she is fourteen years old and is probably demonstrating the normal assertiveness and struggle for independence common to any child of this age. Even if you were her mother, you might well find her demanding and irritating. Understandably, you feel very sensitive about her actions and remarks and are probably inclined to take them personally, although they may not be intended as such. The fact that you think everyone looks at you as if you were a witch does not necessarily mean that that is what they really are thinking. In fact, they may be surprised at your courage in trying to set limits and may be simply recognizing how difficult your situation is (most people in your position would be inclined to be overindulgent in an attempt to ingratiate themselves with their stepdaughter).

Before her next visit, I think it is essential for you to discuss this situation openly and directly with her father. Make it clear to him that you expect her to behave in a courteous and cooperative way while she is in your home and that you would like his help in enforcing certain rules and regulations. If he has any objections or recommendations, iron them out with him beforehand. Once this is done, urge him to talk with his daughter before her next visit to make it clear that he thinks your desires are reasonable. He should convey to the girl the feelings of respect and warmth that you have toward her and explain that he respects and supports your feelings whether he has the same feelings or not.

In this way, the ground rules will be set in advance, and his daughter will know that although she may not like these limits, she is expected to accept them. This will explain any discrepancy between the values her father has previously held and those you wish to enforce now, and at the same time make it clear that your guidelines and wishes are to be accepted.

Is Santa Claus Real?

Every year my neighbor and I get into an argument about Santa Claus: I think it's fun for children to think he exists; she says it's sentimental make-believe that's not good for them. Does she have a point?

I think it is crucially important for parents to be honest with their children, even if the matters concerned seem trivial and harmless to adults.

Making Santa Claus "real" requires many lies. How do you explain all the Santas in all the different stores at Christmas time? How does he get down your chimney when you don't have a fireplace? And most important of all, how do you one day explain that all the answers you gave to all these questions weren't really true,

I believe it is best to tell children that Santa Claus is a make-believe person and that both children and grownups pretend he brings presents at Christmas time. Children are delighted that grownups can engage in make-believe also. In this way, you do not detract from a child's pleasure and you avoid having to tell stories that later may cause a child to doubt your credibility as a parent.

Attachment to Special Toys

I've always discouraged my children from clinging excessively to and going to bed with toys, stuffed animals, and so on, because I don't want them to be too dependent on these things. My children are five and three—and they talk and "party" with their dolls and animals, and at nap and bedtime take along practically every stuffed creature they own. My mother, though, says children need these objects as "comforters," and it's important they have them. Who's right?

I agree with your mother. Children sometimes find great comfort in their stuffed toys. As they go off to sleep, these toys help them make the transition from the waking world into a dream world and give them the reassurance that they are not being detached from everything that is familiar. Moreover, children project many of their feelings and ideas onto their toys and find it comforting to have these "friends" close by to communicate with.

The fantasies of children are delightful, and stuffed animals and toys are objects that allow them to nurture and enact these fantasies. I always loved watching my own young daughter gather stuffed toys around a little table for an afternoon tea party. A child's conversation with these animals provides a means of practicing various social skills, as well as an immediate companionship with friends who have the characteristics that a child wants them to have at that very moment.

The only time a child might grow *too* dependent upon possessions such as these is when the rest of the child's life lacks sufficient stimulation.

More often than not, children give up their dependency on their toys as they grow older—and yet there are many teenagers I know (and even adults) who still enjoy keeping a stuffed object from early childhood. Even this kind of attachment, as unusual as it may be, is not what I call a serious emotional hang-up. Obviously, if a person has many neurotic symptoms accompanying this kind of dependency, then the problem requires professional investigation. However, prohibiting children from having stuffed toys to avoid this possibility will in no way prevent an emotional problem but may in fact cause some transitory discomfort as they face the frustration of being separated from their friendly and reassuring world of stuffed animals.

The Overly Imaginative Child

My husband and I are rather concerned about our three-year-old daughter, Jenny. When we call her by name, she'll say she's not Jenny but Ann and insist that she has red hair and a puppy and a friend named Susan who spills her milk a lot. This has been going on for some months now, and my husband is afraid that this sort of behavior could indicate the start of a split personality. Is this possible? She seems so happy and normal in every other respect.

It is not at all unusual for imaginative children of this age to construct a world of their own filled with the objects and relationships they wonder about. This sort of game gives your daughter an opportunity to try out a different identity—one in which she can test her ability to deal with various fantasy situations and one that she can easily abandon if anything goes wrong. Since your daughter sounds normal and happy in other respects, I think her fantasies are the product of a healthy, creative mind rather than an indication of a schizoid, or split, personality.

If *you*, however, react as if her fantasies are real, this can be very confusing to her. While you must not belittle her imaginary constructions, you must certainly let her know that there is a difference between what she imagines and what is real. If you talk with her in a casual and accepting way about her "pretend" friends, you are showing respect for her feelings and ideas but at the same time establishing an appropriate distinction between what is fantasy and what is reality.

Some children have imaginary companions who supposedly do all the things the children themselves are forbidden to do—"Susan" is the one who ate too many cookies or let the cat into the house. In this way, children are periodically able to show defiance, testing their parents' reactions without, theoretically, jeopardizing themselves. If this is the case, parents should make it clear that the child is responsible for the actions of the imaginary playmate—and this may lead to the abandonment of the make-believe troublemaker.

The Quiet Child

Our four-year-old son seems very happy playing by himself—and we weren't particularly concerned about this until his nursery-school teacher told us that she thought he should be more "social." It's true that he'll sit for long periods of time engrossed with his toys or puzzles. Is it all right for my son to be so much in a world of his own?

I see nothing wrong with a child's being engrossed in his games and even his fantasies as long as he shows a normal capacity to relate to other people when necessary. Many children pass through stages such as this when their activity is more self-play than social interaction; and these same children at other stages of development may become very social and engage in gratifying and meaningful play with others. If your child is *always* in his own world, however, and seems unable to ever interact socially, this may reflect an emotional problem that requires professional help.

A key question is whether your son is able even in his fantasies to maintain a sense of reality. When my own son, Eric, was three and a half, he played by himself a great deal. One day his nursery-school teacher found him staring at a car that he had parked in a toy garage. He sat motionless for such a long time that she finally said, "Eric, wouldn't you like to play with the other children?" He said, "No, I can't. This car is broken and in the garage—I'm waiting for the garage man to fix it." While his teacher was worried that his absorption in fantasy indicated a problem, I was convinced that this was not a problem because even in his fantasies he had a healthy grip on reality: he knew that it takes a long time to have a car fixed.

By the way, the following year a different teacher was concerned because "Eric always plays with other children and rarely plays by himself." Many parents—including myself—often get such reactions from their children's teachers. There is no hard-and-fast rule about the "normal" amount of time a child should spend alone or with others.

Daydreaming

My daughter, almost nine, is a daydreamer. She forgets from one minute to the next what she's been sent to do, forgets to feed the dog or hang up her clothes, and is getting behind in her schoolwork—it has become a problem! Is this something for us to be seriously alarmed about?

Children of this age often engage in daydreaming, and occasional forgetfulness is understandable. However, if she is getting behind in her schoolwork, this may indicate a more serious problem. Perhaps a trip to her school and a discussion with her teachers will help. Is she bored? Is she getting along well with the other children? Does she need help with her schoolwork? These are questions you ought to investigate and talk over with your daughter.

I do not think that your reaction at this time should be one of alarm but one of watchful concern.

Then, if the problem continues, you might consider seeking professional help.

Attachment to Pets

Our six-year-old daughter is more fond of the family cat than she is of us. She spends hours in the yard with the cat and takes it to bed with her at night, talking to it as if it were human. It's as if she didn't know the rest of the world existed. Should we be alarmed?

No, I don't think you should be alarmed. In fact I think you have the wrong interpretation of this situation. I don't think she is *more* fond of the family cat than she is of you. Her fondness for the cat can be intense, but it is not necessarily on the same continuum as her fondness for you. While I wouldn't put the question to her, I bet if she had a choice between her parents or the cat she would pick her parents! Remember, she probably has the security of her family as the stage, or background, for her attachment to the cat. Clearly she is deeply involved with this cat, which is not at all uncommon with children.

Seymour, my daughter's cat, is very much a part of our family and is not only treated humanly but responds accordingly. I'm delighted to see my daughter's expression of love, fondness, and protection of her cat. She sees him as her child and demonstrates what I consider to be the utmost in parental responsibility. She has gone so far as to have relegated me to the position of being a grandparent to her cat, and annually I receive birthday greetings, Father's Day cards, and holiday gifts that are from "Seymour—your grandson."

Having responsibility for a pet not only provides children with the opportunity for taking on a role that prepares them for life's responsibilities, pleasures, and commitments, but it also teaches them sensitivity and helps them try out some of the important experiences that will ultimately be beneficial for their adult human interactions. To me, there is something very beautiful about a child's fondness for animals and the warm response of that animal to the child that leads me to assure you that you have nothing to worry about. Children sometimes acquire an emotional security in a relationship with an animal that they are unable to get in their relationships with people. But, in all likelihood, your child simply has a special relationship with her cat as well as a special relationship with you. If she didn't feel the emotional security and warmth of her relationship with you, she would probably have very little love to offer her cat. Look at it this way: she's showing parental behavior and protectiveness toward her cat that she has probably learned from her own parents' feelings and commitment to her.

Physical Changes in Appearance

My husband was considering shaving off the beard he has had for the past several years—but then it occurred to him that this might be a real shock for our two-year-old. It really made us wonder. Do you think that a change in a parent's appearance could affect a young child's emotional security?

No, I don't think that a physical change such as this would affect your two-year-old. True, he might be temporarily surprised by and curious about his father's new appearance, but if he has a warm and loving relationship with his parents, he will be untouched by almost any kind of physical change a parent undergoes. Do, however, let your son know in advance what your husband intends to do. (And if you have any real apprehension about this, perhaps your two-year-old could even watch as your husband gradually shaves off his beard.)

Children generally accept their parents' appearance in a matter-of-fact way. When my daughter, Pia, was three, she looked at me and said, "Daddy, most men have hair *on* their heads—did yours grow inside your head?" As far as she was concerned, I had hair like most others, and if it was not out in the open where she could readily see it, it simply must be somewhere else.

Nighttime Fears

My five-year-old is obsessed with "witches and mean animals" that she says are hiding in her closet and under her bed. She seems to be genuinely afraid about their being there—and it does no good to try to tease her out of this. Do all children go through a stage of fearing monsters in their rooms at night?

I have known very few children who have not experienced this. Children go through stages where they are frightened by their own hostile and aggressive impulses, particularly if they have not yet learned how to channel them into constructive activity. At times like this children are inclined to project their hostilities onto their environment—saying, in effect, "It's not *me* who's angry; it's something outside of me." In order to make the situation even more tolerable, they tend to displace their aggressions onto frightening creatures or animals. In this way, children are able to express their anger and hostility while simultaneously learning how to cope with this hostility in a socially acceptable way.

As most parents know, reasoning with children about monsters—and even showing them with a flashlight that the monster is *not* there—has hardly any effect. The child's fears are not alleviated, because the actual hostility and the fear of that hostile object originates in the child's mind on an emotional basis and has to be dealt with precisely on that level. It is for this reason that I recommend that parents offer substantial reassurance, and certainly never tease or ridicule. Acknowledge that the child is in fact really frightened of something and that you understand this fear. Obviously, though, if these fears are intense, cause severe panic, and tend to persist, you should definitely seek professional help.

Scary Movies

I find my kids—their ages are five to twelve—enraptured by monster movies on television. I hate the things and some of them scare me, but the kids laugh and seem to love them. Is it harmful for them to be exposed to such frightening and spooky stuff?

Not all young children are enraptured by monster movies. Some are terrified and have horrible nightmares after seeing them. Generally speaking, though, children know how much they can tolerate without feeling intense anxiety. I know of many little children who avoid seeing certain programs on television because they know they will be upsetting for them.

Clearly, monster movies cause a great deal of arousal. Some people feel overwhelmed by this arousal and find it a negative experience, while others find such "horrifying" stimulation to be exciting and enlivening. From a psychological viewpoint, these movies may enable children to drain off their hostile and aggressive feelings. For others who feel anxious about their hostility and aggression, witnessing monster movies and tolerating their own anxiety gives them a sense of mastery—a child may have the feeling "I'm not scared by *that*." (This kind of reaction is not limited to children. How many times have you heard people leaving a movie theater and saying, "That was horrible—I'm glad I didn't miss it!" Some people seem to subject themselves to frightening experiences in a secret attempt to master their anxiety over the very things they fear.

There are, of course, some children in whom such horrifying movies will arouse enough anxiety to intensify their need to remain close to their parents and will even precipitate some regression to immature behavior patterns. This, however, does not seem to be the case with your children. For the most part, I don't think that the monster movies one sees on television are significantly harmful to young minds. I wholeheartedly believe, though, that the television industry could better use the time given to such movies for programs that are not only entertaining but educational and socially useful as well.

Television Violence

Would you please say something about kids and how they are affected by violence on TV? I really wonder when I find my eight-year-old in front of the television set watching programs filled with horror and crime. Does this sort of exposure to brutality affect children?

It is much too easy to hold television responsible for the violence in our country, and I only wish that it were as simple as all that. We would then merely have to eliminate television and movies and all the violence would stop.

On occasion, I am sure that some children have picked up a violent idea from television and acted it out in real life. But such children were prone to expressions of violence in the first place, and television simply reinforced an already existing impulse. I do not think that there is a direct relationship between what children see on a screen and what they do. What does make an impression is how the child's own parents deal with their anger, aggression, and hostility. Children are much more influenced by the people they love and rely on for protection than they are by make-believe characters. If parents go into rages and lash out at others in a cruel and harmful way, children may adopt this as a pattern for their own lives; if parents attempt to communicate their anger in an honest and positive way, and then use their energies to attempt to make things better, a child is bound to be influenced by this, too. Also, if parents help children to gain positive recognition for their worthwhile accomplishments, acts of kindness, or scholarship, children will have less need to achieve recognition through acts of hostility and aggression.

Some professionals even believe that by observing violence on television children are able to discharge hostile feelings of their own. I am inclined to agree. When you stop to think of it, there are violent fairy tales and even religious stories that have persisted for many, many years without harmful effect. Fairy tales such as "Hansel and Gretel" may have made many children anxious and horrified, but they have also provided an acceptable outlet for some of a child's angry feelings and frustrations.

It is important, however, that parents put these scenes of television violence into perspective. When acts of brutality and callousness—whether shown as fiction or as part of a news broadcast—appear on the screen, parents should not merely sit back passively. They should express their feelings of annoyance and disgust at insensitive and cruel actions and thereby give children the reassuring guidelines they need for standards of decent behavior.

Threats About the Boogeyman

My husband told the kids there was a boogeyman in the closet who will eat them up if they don't finish their food. Not only do I think that this is an unfair way to threaten them, but now I have to deal with their belief in a boogeyman. How can I discourage this?

I agree with you, this is an unfair way to treat children. I would go so far as to say it's abusive, deceptive, psychologically damaging, and disrespectful of a child's integrity. Unfortunately, there are many parents who threaten their children with a boogeyman or its equivalent. Children are trusting until parents prove themselves untrustworthy. Theats of this sort are one way of damaging that trust.

The best way to discourage this is by insisting that your husband stop these threats. Let him know how damaging it can be to his children's relationship with him. The best way of helping the children at this point is to get your husband to confront them with his having deceived them. If he tells them he made up the story of the boogeyman and is sorry that he did, if he lets them know that he actually wanted to help them eat their meals better but now realizes it was unfair of him to do it this way, the children may regain their trust in him and abandon their fear of the boogeyman.

I truly believe that parents should always be honest with their children. Some parents feel the end justifies the means. They think if they can get a child to do what they want, even by deception, they are "good parents." While the parent may gain in the short term, in the long run the damage it can do to a trusting relationship far outweighs any short-term advantages. Apart from the inherent indignities this kind of threat is to a child, it is precisely the distrust it breeds that causes children to turn to their peers and to other authorities more extensively than to their own parents when they have questions or concerns about life's problems.

Frightening Bedtime Stories

My husband insists on telling frightening stories to the children at dinner time. They love it until bedtime, when they're too frightened to sleep and want to get into bed with us. My husband thinks it's funny, but I'm not getting any sleep. What should I do?

I think you should tell your husband to stop telling frightening stories to your children at dinner time. I'm sure he enjoys the children's amusement at his storytelling, but it's not at all amusing if they are deprived of their sleep. I believe your children's amusement lies not in the frightening nature of the stories but in the fact that their father actively participates with them in conversation at dinner time and tells them detailed stories. I am sure that if the content of the stories changes, the problem will be solved. It's important to remember, and I repeat, that the pleasure your children receive is not built around the frightening nature of the stories, but the fact that your husband shows his enthusiasm in his involvement with them. Perhaps you should suggest to your husband that he try to tell stories that are amusing, exciting, and filled with anticipation, yet lack the element of fear that seems to disturb your children.

Fear of the Dark

Our twelve-year-old daughter has been afraid of the dark all her life and doesn't show any signs of growing out of this problem. She sleeps with the light on in her bedroom and doesn't dare go into the cellar or upstairs to the attic by herself. Is this unusual? Is there anything we can do to help her overcome her fear?

This is not at all unusual. In fact, it's common. Understandably, it's frightening to children to be in the dark—and, for that matter, all people as they advance along in life seem to carry with them some degree of fear of the dark. Darkness is considered sinister, and throughout adult life we use expressions that associate darkness with mystery, danger, the unknown, and evil. At the same time, we tend to think of bravery as being associated with the ability to forge ahead into the darkness without any fear whatsoever. Anyone who ventures into the darkness or the unknown carries with him or her some degree of anxiety. The fact that some persons can have control over anxiety and perhaps still be able to deal with the unknown does not mean they didn't have some fear of the dark in the first place. I venture to say that most adults have some trepidations about going into a cellar or into an attic unaccompanied. This, in my mind, does not reflect an emotional problem; it shows some respect for the uncertainties that exist in life.

If your daughter is a generally fearful child, has trouble getting along with other children, shows difficulty in school, and shows other signs of being overwhelmed by uncertainty to the degree that it prevents her from functioning in everyday life, I would then suggest that you seek some professional guidance initially for diagnosing her condition and secondarily to see if treatment for her behavior is appropriate.

Nightmares

My two-year-old has nightmares—he wakes up during the night sobbing and frightened. But since he can't verbalize his dreams, I'm at a loss as to what is causing them. Is it natural for such small children to have nightmares?

It is very common for children of this age to have occasional nightmares—ones that are intensely frightening because they arouse their fear of abandonment by parents or others whose protection is needed to maintain their emotional security. It is at these moments that frightened children especially need to be helped and reassured of your love.

Many nightmares of children this age are filled with monsters, scary people, animals, and sometimes machinery and other things that are dangerous and uncontrollable. Dreams are, in a sense, a construction of a child's own mind. Two-year-old children normally go through a stage in which they are hostile, aggressive, and negativistic, and they will often displace or transfer these impulses onto those "terrifying" things in their dreams. These nightmares often represent the struggle within children to come to terms with their own hostile, and aggressive impulses that they have not yet mastered. As time passes and some of these fears are resolved, your child's dreams will take other forms, but as long as you are there to offer comfort and support, these nightmares should have no disturbing effect on your child's development.

The Clinging Child and Separation

My fourteen-month-old daughter seems to find it impossible to entertain herself alone for even five minutes. I play with her throughout the day, but the minute I leave to try to fix supper or answer the phone, she starts screaming and will not stop. What should I do?

Children vary in their need for parental attention, but the child who clings the most probably has some fear of abandonment. Most fourteen-month-old children *are* able to play by themselves for longer periods of time, and the fact that your daughter screams so emphatically when left alone could be a message that she fears you will not return—ever.

This sort of reaction may be due to frightening experiences perpetrated by well-meaning adults.

For instance, a parent with all good intentions may put a child to sleep, have a strange babysitter come to the house, and then go off to a movie. The child awakens, sees an unfamiliar person, and feels panic. A few occasions like this and a child becomes desperate to have a parent near at all times.

Perhaps the best way to deal with your daughter's distress is to get her partly involved in what you are doing while preparing dinner, or to keep her close to you in spite of the inconvenience it causes at the moment. As time passes, she should be substantially reassured that letting you out of sight does not mean letting you out of her life altogether.

My fifteen-month-old son is painfully shy, and very clingy. Recently, we took him to a party of children his own age, and while the others toddled and enjoyed themselves, he stayed in his daddy's arms the whole time. Should we just wait for him to grow out of this or should we attempt to force him out into social situations?

I do not think you should attempt to force him out into social situations. This will only serve to inhibit him more and make him cling more intently. For reasons of his own, he is overwhelmed by these situations and feels greater security in his daddy's arms. Remember, he is only fifteen months of age, and children this age are not really ready to socialize with other children. Often they simply enjoy being on the outside, observing what is taking place. I have seen innumerable parents who complain of shyness in their children during the first few years of life; after determining that there was no deep-rooted emotional problem or fear of separation, I urged them to wait it out and not force their children. Quite spontaneously, the child emerged into a more social being around the age of three or four—with some children not until five—and all traces of shyness subsided. Recently, I was discussing this very problem with the director of our nursery school at The New York Hospital, a person I greatly admire. She recounted an episode of a three-year-old she knew who was quite shy, whose shyness was tolerated. When this three-year-old became a four-year-old she seemed more outgoing and her shyness subsided. When she was told by our nursery-school director, "You seem to have overcome your shyness—how come?" She replied, "People seem to be getting friendlier and friendlier." This not only attests to the fact that children often overcome the problem spontaneously, but it also tells you that children respond to the world in terms of their own feelings about themselves.

Being Afraid of Babysitters

My child has never gotten used to the arrival of a babysitter. She starts to wail the moment someone walks into the house, whether she knows the babysitter already or whether it is a stranger. I can't bear the agony. What can I do to help her and yet allow myself some free time?

A child will frequently show an inordinate amount of fear of a babysitter if, at some time, the parents have put the child to sleep before a babysitter came and left without the child's knowing it. If that child awakens while the parents are gone and finds a stranger there, it cannot only be terribly frightening to a child but can create terrible sleep problems later on. A little child may interpret the parents' going away and a stranger appearing as having been caused by going to sleep in the first place. While this may seem illogical to an adult, it is consistent with the child's interpretation of reality.

A child will also show undue distress at the sight of a babysitter if that child has had unpleasant experiences with a babysitter in the past. With all due respect to babysitters, I've known of many situations where a child has fallen, has been ignored, or has been directly terrorized by a babysitter in the course of a parent's absence. Frequently these events do not come to the attention of the parents but may manifest themselves by an intense fear on the part of the child when any babysitter appears. I've also noticed that some children show an intense aversion to babysitters if their parents have gone off for days at a time before the child has gotten to understand the concept of today, tomorrow, and the next day and has therefore been deprived of any preparation for a prolonged parental excursion away from home. Children who have had this experience under the age of two or two and a half frequently become terrified that each time a babysitter arrives it means the parents will go away for an indefinite period.

Regardless of what has caused your child's intense reactions, I think you should pick perhaps two or three babysitters who are warm and friendly and who truly enjoy children. You can best judge this by watching them handle your child. If you have confidence in them, in all likelihood your child will eventually feel similarly. Have these people come and play with your child while you are home for perhaps an hour or two at a time. Eventually, your child can establish a positive relationship with these sitters and interpret their visits as playful times. It will not only help your child establish a positive relationship with the sitter, but it will also give you a chance to observe that person as your surrogate when you will eventually be gone. After your child has gotten used to these sitters and no longer reacts to their arrival as the equivalent of your disappearance, you can then begin to leave for short periods of time, which can then be extended to give you the free time you need.

While this may seem like a tedious process to go through, it will have long-range benefits and will serve to help your child master her fears of those strangers she interprets as a threat to the integrity of her relationship with you.

The Clinging Child

Whenever I try to leave my three-year-old son with anyone, he cries frantically and hangs on to me, and for this reason I seldom go any place without him. How is it best to break him of this pattern?

It is not usual for a three-year-old to cry frantically and cling to a parent in this way unless he has had some unpleasant experience involving separation from you. If parents are careful to prepare children gradually for this and if they avoid frequent separations when their children are very young, it is unlikely that such a pattern will develop.

As I have mentioned before, I find that many parents put their small children to sleep, have a strange babysitter come, and then "sneak out" for an evening at the movies. On their return, they find a panic-stricken child who not only clings to both parents but becomes fearful that going to sleep causes the parents to go away.

I think it is important to introduce babysitters gradually during the first year of a child's life so that he realizes that other people can care for him adequately when his own parents are not around. However, make sure that your child knows that you are leaving, reassure him that you will return, and do not make the initial separations longer than a few hours. It is best if you maintain the same two or three familiar people as babysitters.

If your child cannot be separated from you without crying indefinitely, you may need to seek professional help to gain insight into your specific situation. Often, though, children get over this problem spontaneously if their parents do not engage in tactics to fool the child while they slip away, or make false promises of gifts or events that might occur if the child will let them go.

Summer Camp and the Reluctant Child

Our daughter is eleven and shy for her age. My husband thinks it would do wonders for her to go away to a summer camp (we've heard about an excellent one) for a month. But although she's slept overnight with friends, she's never been away from home for any longer than that—and she's very unhappy about the prospect of going so far away from home for so long a time. I agree with my husband that such an experience would be good for her, but I hate to insist that she go if she really doesn't want to. Do you think we should make her go "for her own good"?

Your daughter may be shy but she doesn't sound overly apprehensive. If she's able to spend an occasional night with friends without anxiety, she's obviously capable of handling periodic separations. But while camp can be a rewarding experience, there are some children who prefer more family-oriented situations. The fact that she is unhappy about the thought of going away may simply reflect her sincere desire to be with her family.

If she does not want to go to camp, do not insist she do so. This not only would make her resentful but could force her into a situation that might create sufficient anxiety to interfere with her growing independence. Let this independence emerge with your encouragement, but don't insist she take a long stint away from home until she is ready.

You might find it helpful to have your daughter *visit* a summer camp, simply to get a more realistic idea of what it's like there. Perhaps in the course of your summer vacation you can plan such a trip, and this would give you all a better perspective from which to organize subsequent summers—and give your daughter the option of deciding on her own whether this is what she wants next year.

Anxieties with Sleep-Away Visits

My six-year-old has spent overnights with her little friends and when she was invited to go away for an entire week of vacation with them, she looked forward to it excitedly. But the very first night we received a call from the seashore—she was sobbing and begging to come home. Even though it was a very long drive, we drove there the next day to bring her home, but I'm not convinced we did the right thing to go running. Would it have been better if we insisted she stick the visit out?

No. You did the right thing by responding to her anxiety and fear. Remember she is only a six-year-old and still needs a great deal of parental protection and help in dealing with the things she fears. Had your daughter been ten or eleven years of age, it might have been wiser to have her stick it out, but at this age she needed your help. It is quite common for children this age to become enthusiastic about a visit such as this before it actually takes place. It represents "growing up" and "independence," and in her fantasy about the trip everything was fine. Nevertheless, when the reality took place and she was actually away from her family things obviously looked quite different. Something must have triggered anxiety, and she found no one there with the same degree of concern for her feelings that her own parents had.

When you pick her up, you should reassure her that she tried, and even though it didn't work out this time, perhaps it will the next time. In this way you show recognition of her fears and respect for her feelings and avoid having her see this experience as a failure.

As a general rule, when parents prepare children for separations such as this, it is wise to let them know in advance that it may not work out and that they may feel homesickness.

If you approach a situation like this with understanding, your child is likely to tell you what it is that caused her fear to become so intense that she had to come home. If you have this kind of relationship with your child and she feels capable of expressing her feelings, you can help her more effectively in dealing with her separation anxiety than if you tease her, make fun of her, or give her feelings of failure. Let her know you will give her all the support she needs the next time she plans a visit away, and perhaps you can make it a shorter visit and less challenging.

Visits Away from Home

My parents would like to keep our year-old daughter for a week this summer. Is a child of this age too young to be away from her mother and father for this length of time?

Children of this age are still very much dependent upon their own parents. They also do not have a concept of time that enables them to know the difference between "now" and "a week from now," and it may seem to them that they have been permanently abandoned. I have seen many children react to such visits by later showing an increase in dependent behavior; sometimes they experience sleep problems and occasionally may seem unattached to their own parents.

Sometimes such visits are a necessity, and in many instances they seem to cause no problems at all. But, if possible, I think it best to put off such prolonged visits until your child is perhaps two or two and a half. At that time, your daughter will understand how long a week is and will be better able to realize that you *will* return to take her home.

Problems for the Traveling Parent

I am a divorcee and a working mother, and my nine-year-old daughter seems intent on making each of my periodic business trips a heartrending experience. All the details concerning my trips are explained to her, and the babysitting arrangements are excellent. Yet, she insists on tear-filled scenes, and my departures are punctuated with racking sobs. How do I deal with what has become an awful problem when I actually must depart?

Frankly, I would be more concerned if your nine-year-old showed no reaction at all or seemed happy at the time of your leaving. It is natural for a child who understandably depends on a parent for love, support, and protection to have an emotional reaction when a separation is taking place. No matter how excellent the babysitting arrangements are, your daughter wants *you* and feels vulnerable when you are not there. If you have not already tried spending extra time with her prior to these trips, do so. Perhaps you can give her more individual attention for two or three days prior to a trip, taking her to a restaurant or movie alone to affirm your desire to be with her. Telephone her each day while you are gone and let her know that you miss her and are thinking about her. Find something you know she would like as a gift, so she knows you went out of your way for her.

Having two parents who are very busy with little time for their children usually creates some problems; having one busy parent who also must be away from home altogether for periods of time makes the situation even more difficult for the child. If she can be with her father during these times that you are gone or if you can perhaps take her on these trips with you periodically, you will be diminishing the amount of time she would be spending away from both her parents at the same time.

Lack of Self-Reliance

My children are both completely lost if they come home from school one afternoon without a date with a friend or an organized activity to go to. How can I teach my children to be more self-reliant and depend less on others to provide entertainment?

I don't think you should look upon your children's behavior as lacking self-reliance or being overly dependent on others. It sounds as if they are very social and enjoy sharing their time with friends. Some children are more social than others. Also, all children go through phases and fluctuate between group-oriented activities and individual activities. And it's important for parents to recognize that some children seem to be more ingenious in their ability to find things to occupy themselves with alone. Carried to an extreme however, your child can become so self-sufficient that he not only doesn't need other people but could actually shy away from them and become what we call a "loner."

Perhaps you can get your children interested in some activities such as model building or reading or some other activity that can be engaged in alone. While interesting your children in individual activities, be careful not to convey the idea that there's anything wrong with wanting to have playmates or relying upon them for companionship. It's far better for children in the long run when parents can stress individual differences, pointing out that some people have a tendency to prefer individual activities while other people tend to want to do things with others. If you accept both as normal, your child will not only have a greater sense of self-esteem but will also be inclined to be more accepting of all people regardless of their differences. Attempts to make a child feel that there is one right way and all other ways are wrong serves to make them intolerant of different social, racial, religious, and physical differences they see among human beings.

Vacations Away from Your Child

My husband and I really need a vacation when we can be alone for a week or so, but we are concerned about the emotional effect that our absence might have on our eight-month-old son. We'd be leaving him with his grandparents—he's familiar with them and they get along very well—but we wonder if this separation will have any effect on him.

You are fortunate that your child knows his grandparents and gets along well with them. This will indeed make the separation more bearable. However, when parents go off for a week or more, it is common for little children to become very attached to their "caretakers." When parents return, they are often dismayed because their child turns away from them and seems to prefer the grandparents, the babysitter, or whoever was present during their absence. This tendency of a baby to grow attached to others may be something of a shock to parents who had not expected it.

In some instances, children of this age become

depressed while the parents are gone and may even stop eating. In many cases, children also develop sleep problems, which may persist even after the parents return. Nor is it surprising for little children to have temper tantrums and indulge in destructive behavior following a parental separation. Often they will cling a great deal and find it hard to allow the returned parents out of their sight for any length of time. These reactions may occur because it is difficult for a child under the age of two to understand that even though the parents have gone away, they *will* eventually return. And when the parents are once again close by, children may need a great deal of reassurance that they will not go away again.

I am not suggesting that you and your husband cancel the needed vacation. But I think it is essential for you to be prepared for and understand the problems you may encounter, so that you will be able to deal intelligently with any symptoms that may occur during your trip and after your return.

The Intellectually Curious Toddler

My twenty-two-month-old son seems exceptionally bright. He knows all the letters of the alphabet and some words associated with them—and because he is quick to remember and eager to learn, I find it hard not to teach him new things. Now friends have advised us that we may be causing problems for him when he starts school later. What do you think?

I find that for some strange reason most parents assume that *other* people are correct in cases like this. But not all the advice given by friends and relatives is objective or in a child's best interest. In fact, a great deal of this advice only serves to undermine parents' natural protective tendencies and their confidence in doing what they feel is best.

As long as you maintain a warm and supportive relationship with your twenty-two-month-old and do not transform your role as a parent into that of a teacher, I see no harm whatsoever in your responding to his curiosity in this way. If you provide him with the materials and the stimulation he needs, it is likely that his quest for new knowledge will continue, and this may lead to greater intellectual achievement later on. It sounds to me as if your friends are telling you to stunt his intellectual curiosity so that he will be like an average child. If, in fact, he is showing intellectual precociousness, he may need a particularly stimulating academic environment when he starts school, but to suggest that you retard his intellectual development at this point seems not only absurd but very risky. To do so could cause him so much frustration that he might become angry, defiant, and closed to possibilities for growth in the future. Take care of his needs at *this* stage in his development, and when he is ready to go to school, deal with that situation in a manner that is appropriate to his capacities and interests at that time.

Problems with Music Lessons and Practicing

My eleven-year-old daughter has been taking piano lessons for a year or so now, and we've gotten into a real battle about practicing. My daughter resists, I insist, she winds up in tears. I've often wished my parents had made me practice so I could play the piano now.

How adamant should parents be about insisting that their children play a musical instrument?

I do not think parents should be adamant at all about having their children take music lessons. Instead, parents should attempt to provide their children with a stimulating and rich environment and give them the opportunity to pursue their own interests and desires.

If your child *is* musically inclined and wishes to take lessons, there are obviously certain responsibilities that should be clear—one of which involves caring for the instrument itself; another is actually practicing on the instrument. But constant insistence that a child practice will create conflict, and soon the child will associate music with a feeling of unpleasantness. Perhaps a more flexible attitude on your part is the answer. Talk with your daughter about whether she really wishes to learn to play the piano, and if she does, explain that her desire involves a certain amount of commitment on her part. If the time or the duration of the practice sessions seems restrictive to her, perhaps you could plan them for another hour, or at shorter intervals throughout the day.

But it is unfair for you to impose frustrations from your own childhood on your daughter. If *you* still have the desire to play the piano now, why not take lessons yourself? You might find a renewed interest on your daughter's part if she saw her mother enjoying music lessons and the satisfaction that practice brings.

I received a call from my fourteen-year-old son's teacher, who said that my son had been caught cheating on a math exam. I was horrified—and also mystified, since he's a fairly good student. He was very casual when we confronted him and said, "Oh, I didn't know the answer and just looked at Tommy's paper." My husband and I were embarrassed and so we let it drop for the moment, but it's really on our minds. How should we deal with this? Why do kids who are bright and capable cheat?

You should never drop a problem like this or pretend it didn't happen. It should certainly be discussed with your son in a serious and concerned manner. Do not be punitive with him or harp on the fact that it was "embarrassing" to you and your husband. After all, that's your problem and not his. The primary point for discussion is the fact that he knowingly cheated, which is *wrong*. It is important for all people to feel a sense of guilt if they cheat or steal or lie. If they simply feel there is nothing wrong with such behavior—"as long as you don't get caught"—they lack the proper values that mold behavior in a socially acceptable manner. In recent years I have been appalled at the number of times I had heard well-known people in government justify dishonesty by saying "everyone does it." When values like this are transmitted to our youth, it leads to a weakening in the conscience of people and implies that success means getting away with things that are unearned.

I think your son should know your deep concern about this. Let him know that this kind of behavior can get him into a great deal of trouble. Emphasize the importance of honesty and effort in doing his own work and building his sense of personal worth. Talk about the fact that a grade is simply an evaluation of what he has learned and should not be his primary goal. Make it clear that "just looking at Tommy's paper" was not simply "just looking" but cheating.

In all likelihood, this is an isolated event for you. However, if it continues, your son may be having some underlying emotional problem, of which his cheating is a symptom. Sometimes children who are angry with their parents but unable to express it verbally do so by getting into the kind of trouble that is in fact embarrassing to their parents or causes their parents some form of suffering. Face up to this problem and attempt to discuss it with your son. By dropping the issue, you are in a sense condoning his behavior passively. Or, if it is due to some underlying resentment toward you, you may be forcing him to do something even more horrendous as a means of expressing his anger.

Feigning Sickness to Avoid School

My ten-year-old has recently begun pretending to be sick so that I will let her stay home with me rather than going to school. She has a perfectly wonderful teacher, who reports no academic or behavior problems in the classroom and is baffled by this situation as much as I am. Should I force her to go to school or let her stay home where she wants?

You have to establish some ground rules for this situation. It's impossible to call a doctor each morning your child complains of sickness to establish whether she is in fact sick. At the same time you need some criterion by which to judge the seriousness of the situation. I believe you should take your child's temperature, and if there is no fever or other definite symptoms, she should go to school. At the same time, let your child know that everyone has days when he or she would rather do something other than what is required, but it's necessary to pull yourself together and do what you are supposed to do anyway. Let her know school is one of her responsibilities and that she simply can't arbitrarily decide she doesn't want to go.

Since she has no difficulties in school, perhaps there are concerns she has about home that make her want to be there. I've found that when family problems arise and there is uncertainty about the future of a family, children frequently want to stay at home for fear that something will happen and they will be abandoned. If this is not the case in your family and you find no reason to believe that she has anxieties about home that cause her to want to be there, you might consider the possibility that she is bored in school and is attempting to manipulate you into letting her stay at home, which she finds more enjoyable than being in school. Under no circumstances should you allow feigned illness to be used to protect her from less pleasant circumstances. This tends to reinforce a pattern where a person uses his or her health to avoid unpleasant situations.

Reacting to Report Cards

Whenever our children bring home their report cards—they're in junior high and high school now—my husband scrutinizes the low marks and chastises the kids for not doing better; sometimes they are even reduced to tears over the whole thing. Do you agree with my husband's tactics? I can't say the children's grades are better because of it.

No, I do not agree with your husband's tactics at all. While I believe strongly in encouraging children to overcome their weaknesses, I am asbolutely against chastising them—especially to the point of tears. Such rebukes cause intense anxiety, threaten your children's sense of self-esteem, and create negative feelings about learning in general.

If school is looked upon merely as a means of achieving grades to "satisfy father," your children will not have that sense of satisfaction and accomplishment that comes from learning for its own sake. Try to get your husband to show positive recognition for the good grades, and both of you do what you can to help the children improve their bad marks. But under no circumstances should your husband emphasize their liabilities and ignore their assets. As you can see, his tactics have not in any way helped—and have doubtless caused your children to feel rejected and resentful.

Avoiding Home Work

My kids (they're eleven and thirteen) hate to do their homework—and when they finally do it, they're so begrudging and half-hearted about it that I wonder if they're learning anything. Does homework do any good, and is it normal for children to dislike it so much?

It is very common for children to deal with their homework in the manner you describe. If you look at it from your children's point of view, they spend a considerable part of each day in school in a fairly organized and regimented schedule, and they are usually bursting with suppressed energies when they leave the classroom at the end of the day. To children, homework is a great obstacle to them at a time when they want and need their freedom and an opportunity to express themselves and to share in family activities.

Let me say this: I am not absolutely against homework, but I certainly think parents and teachers should take a serious look at its actual value. Often the work is a repetition of what students have already done that day in school; it is "busy work," which simply takes time to do and provides little or no educational value. But what concerns me most about uninspiring homework given in large quantities is that it causes children to view school as an unpleasant and tedious place and the educational process an obstacle to their self-expression and the development of their individuality.

I have discussed the matter of homework with many educators and have found that they share my views. But they are under pressure from parents, who often will not consider a school a good school unless their children are given extensive homework assignments.

I would much prefer to see homework assignments that provide children with an opportunity to explore areas that are of particular interest to them. Many children are deeply concerned about ecology, plant life, and animal behavior. Wouldn't it be nice if homework assignments were worked out as projects that would give children an opportunity to broaden their knowledge in these areas? This not only would be more emotionally and intellectually satisfying, but would also teach children how to apply the resources and tools they've learned in school to extend the horizons of their knowledge in the everyday world.

Escape into Books

My son always has his head in a book. I like him to read, but I am getting worried because he never seems to hear us when we talk to him or ask him to do something. Is he using books to hide from all his other responsibilities?

It sounds to me as if he's deeply engrossed in what he's reading and finds it difficult to shift his attention from his book to what you're telling him. I think it's marvelous when children can enjoy books and become engrossed in them. Most parents complain that their children show less interest in books than they'd like them to and frequently complain that their children seem more engrossed in television than in books. Perhaps your child has discovered the world of reading and enjoys his immersion in that world at the present time.

This does not necessarily mean that he's hiding or using it to avoid responsibilities; that depends upon other aspects of his behavior. If he enjoys his friendships, speaks to people about what he's reading, is free of fears and anxieties, and does not appear sullen, morose, or depressed, in all likelihood he is not using it defensively. If, however, he is totally oblivious to everything going on around him and seems to be living out the stories in his books and showing no interest in his own personal hygiene or care, they may reflect an underlying emotional problem for which you should seek psychological help. In evaluating the possibility that a child's behavior pattern represents a problem, it's important to take into consideration all other aspects of the child's behavior and personality rather than to view one symptom as reflective of a serious emotional disorder.

High Motivation—but Low Grades

My child is terribly eager to get good grades in school, but no matter how hard she tries she comes home with C's and is not satisfied with them. What should we do?

Perhaps you should speak with her teacher and let her know how eager your daughter is to get good grades and that you feel she is trying very, very hard to accomplish this. You might also consider discussing the possibility of tutorial help. Conceivably, your daughter is in a class where the children are very competitive and where she feels left out unless her academic achievement is at a higher level. Let your daughter know how pleased you are with her eagerness to do well at school and that you are proud of her efforts. Make it clear that it's not essential for people to be the best in everything but that you consider it important for a person to try hard. Let her know she's doing this and that you admire her for it.

You might also consider the possibility that she is in the wrong school. I've known many children over the years who were deeply distressed by their inability to achieve above an average level and who interpreted this as failure. While I don't believe that parents should move a child from school to school without careful consideration, many of the children I've just described have done extremely well in other schools and found both their educational experience and their social life far more suitable to their own capacities and work style.

It's highly unfortunate for a child who is as well motivated as your daughter to have a sense of failure about school. If these feelings persist for any length of time, or if circumstances are not modified to help her achieve more success, you run the risk of having her lose confidence and perhaps decide, "What's the use—no matter how hard I try I can't succeed." While her motivation is high, do what you can to work the problem out, but by all means involve her in the decisions and give her emotional support while solving the problems.

Dropping Out of School

My son is in his senior year of high school and has always been a good student. But he has just announced that he has no intention of going on to college. He says he wants to get a job in a local filling station and work as a mechanic "until he gets his head together." My husband and I are heartbroken. How can we make him continue his education?

The fact is that many people gain great personal satisfaction and make substantial contributions to society without ever acquiring a formal education. However, rather than rejecting a college education altogether, it seems as if your son is simply not quite sure at this time of what he ultimately wants to do. If he wants to "get his head together," he obviously has some insight and a feeling of seriousness about the future. By working for a while as a mechanic, he probably hopes to gain experience and maturity that will ultimately help him make his decision about the years ahead.

Your son may find that working in a filling station does not come up to the expectations he has about this sort of "simple" life, but the only way for him to find out is to try. If you prevent him from doing what he wants to do, he will always regret not having the experience. The fantasy of "what might have been" will always be with him, and he will resent being pushed onto a path he did not choose.

I'm sorry to say that if you and your husband are heartbroken, it is your problem not your son's. It would not make you happy, I'm sure, to know he was going to school or living his life simply to please you—rather than becoming a happy human being who is achieving his own independence and sense of fulfillment.

Sharing Religion with Children

Both my husband and I are devout Catholics and attend Mass regularly. We feel we should bring up our small children accordingly but wonder, with all the changes going on in the Church, if it would be better to let them decide on a faith later on?

I believe that children should share in all family events, and religious events are no exception. If family events such as church attendance are pleasant and enjoyable and involve respect for the curiosity children have as well as their individuality, they can be positive experiences.

Religion can be a very frightening thing to children, or it can be a very gratifying and organizing concept. It's important for all parents to recognize this, since many parents I know focus on the negative aspects of religious beliefs, such as "going to Hell" or punishment for wrong-doing. A good deal of religion is built around understanding and love and humanity. If people focused more on those factors in each religion that bring people closer together, rather than on the differences that force them apart, any religious belief can serve a very positive purpose for unifying a family and providing a structure for the development of one's beliefs and ideas.

The fact that changes are taking place in the Church and, in all likelihood, will continue as time goes on does not mean that you as a family should not enjoy attending religious ceremonies now. If you truly believe that your children should have the freedom to make their own choices later on regarding religious faith, there is no reason whatsoever why you cannot tell them that now, but indicate what you and your husband believe in and ask them to share in your own customs. I can tell you, out of experience, that they will make their own decisions later on whether you want them to or not. However, unquestionably, their experiences in childhood have a tremendous impact on what their beliefs will be later on. I cannot help but admire your wish to give your children the freedom of choice later on, even though your own beliefs are very clear and devout.

My nine-year-old son refuses to go to Sunday school. We feel that religious schooling and Confirmation are very important. What should we do?

I think you should begin by asking him why he refuses to go. There has to be at least one reason why he feels this way. Not until you uncover his actual reasons will you be in any position to change his mind. Some children find Sunday school too restrictive, particularly if the focus of their religious education is negative and if the teacher tends to be threatening and overbearing. Children spend a good deal of their week attending formal classes and need some time for themselves. Perhaps your child is overburdened with organized after-school activities, like music lessons or additional tutoring, which might make him rebel against additional organized education on Sundays. Whatever his reasons are, it's important for you to get them out into the open where you can discuss them.

I don't think you will accomplish very much by insisting that he attend Sunday school. That would only serve to turn him against your religious beliefs and the idea of Confirmation. I know many children whose parents forced them to go to Sunday school and to receive Confirmation who couldn't wait to get it over with and have simply been turned off when it comes to any of their parents' religious ideas or celebrations. I do think, however, that it's fair for you to insist that he try Sunday school for a period of time before refusing to go. By discussing the matter with him you may find that his arguments are sufficiently convincing for you to put off the idea of Sunday school for perhaps another year.

On the other hand, by taking a compromising attitude and respecting his wishes and feelings in the matter, you might find that after a trial period at Sunday school he finds it sufficiently rewarding to want to continue on his own. Forcing a child or anyone else for that matter to do something he or she doesn't want to do, instead of exploring their reasons for it, invariably leads to resentment, defiance, and rebellion.

About the Author

Dr. Lee Salk is perhaps the best-known child psychologist in America today, honored in his profession and admired by a large popular following for his ability to offer useful advice in a clear and helpful manner.

Dr. Salk currently serves as Clinical Professor of Psychology in Pediatrics and Psychiatry at Cornell University Medical College and is on the staff of the Payne Whitney Psychiatric Clinic of the New York Hospital and in the Pediatrics Department of the Lenox Hill Hospital. He has served as president of both the American Psychological Association's section on Clinical Child Psychology and the Society of Pediatric Psychology.

His monthly column, "You and Your Family," appears in *McCalls* and is one of its most popular features, with a readership of 15 million people. He also has a syndicated weekly newspaper column.

Dr. Salk has appeared extensively on radio and television. He is the author of *How to Raise a Human Being, What Every Child Would Like His Parents to Know* (a national bestseller, subsequently translated into sixteen languages), and *Preparing for Parenthood.*

Among other awards, he has received the Distinguished Contribution Awards from the Society of Pediatric Psychology and the Clinical Child Psychology section of the American Psychological Association. He also received the Pearl Merrill Award "in recognition of his distinguished contribution to the field of Pediatric Psychology and for his warm understanding of the needs of the human family."

Index

MORE HELPFUL BOOKS FROM WARNER...

BE YOUNG WITH YOGA
by Richard L. Hittleman *(89-432, $1.95)*

Looking for good health and the energy of youth? Discover how a few minutes of Yoga will do more for you than hours of ordinary exercise! One of America's foremost Yoga instructors has organized 20 simple yoga techniques into an easy-to-follow, seven week course that will show you how to BE YOUNG WITH YOGA — and never feel old again!

A HANDBOOK OF YOGA FOR MODERN LIVING
by Eugene S. Rawls *(89-596, $1.95)*

Your entire family can follow the Yoga disciplines together. There are back-breaking exercises — instead, you enjoy the gentle, relaxed stretching of muscles and learn how to breathe properly. Begin to use this dynamic new approach to self-development today! The definitive guidebook to health and happiness for everyone in the entire family. Fully illustrated.

YOGA FOR BEAUTY AND HEALTH
by Eugene Rawls and Eve Diskin *(82-972, $2.25)*

Become more alive, more confident, serene and attractive — burst with energy and ambition as you follow the proved teachings of Eugene Rawls and Eve Diskin, two of America's most famous and expert Yoga instructors. Give new youth to your face and body with a modern method that is 4,000 years old! Fully illustrated with step-by-step instructions.

YOGA FOR PHYSICAL FITNESS
by Richard L. Hittleman *(89-099, $1.95)*

Enjoy vibrant good health and sparkling energy with this effective program geared for those whose work prevents them from getting enough exercise. Learn to stimulate circulation, improve muscle tone, eliminate headaches and more. Fully illustrated.

YOGA FOR PERSONAL LIVING
by Richard L. Hittleman *(91-186, $2.50)*

Ten minutes of Yoga practiced in the morning (starting out while still in bed) sets of exhilarating mental and emotional tone for the entire day. Ten minutes of Yoga before going to bed improves skin tone and hair luster, creates a suppler, healthier body, and prepares the way for deep, restful sleep. In YOGA FOR PERSONAL LIVING, Richard L. Hittleman has created a practical guide for everyone.